# A HANDBOOK FOR
# STUDENT NURSES

# HEALTH AND SOCIAL CARE TITLES AVAILABLE FROM LANTERN PUBLISHING LTD

| ISBN | Title |
|---|---|
| 9781906052041 | Clinical Skills for Student Nurses |
| 9781906052065 | Communication and Interpersonal Skills |
| 9781906052027 | Effective Management in Long-term Care Organisations |
| 9781906052140 | Essential Study Skills for Health and Social Care |
| 9781906052171 | First Health and Social Care |
| 9781906052102 | Fundamentals of Diagnostic Imaging |
| 9781906052133 | Fundamentals of Nursing Care |
| 9781906052119 | Improving Students' Motivation to Study |
| 9781906052188 | Interpersonal Skills for the People Professions |
| 9781906052096 | Neonatal Care |
| 9781906052072 | Numeracy, Clinical Calculations and Basic Statistics |
| 9781906052164 | Palliative Care |
| 9781906052201 | Professional Practice in Public Health |
| 9781906052089 | Safe & Clean Care |
| 9781906052157 | The Care and Wellbeing of Older People |
| 9781906052225 | The Care Process |
| 9781906052218 | Understanding and Helping People in Crisis |
| 9781906052010 | Understanding Research and Evidence-Based Practice |
| 9781906052058 | Values for Care Practice |

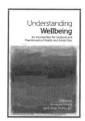

9781908625007

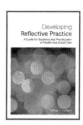

9781908625014

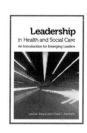

9781908625021

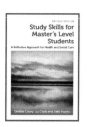

9781908625175

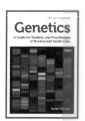

9781908625151

# A HANDBOOK FOR
# STUDENT NURSES

## INTRODUCING KEY ISSUES RELEVANT FOR PRACTICE

### 2ND EDITION

## WENDY BENBOW AND GILL JORDAN

ISBN: 978 1 908625 14 4
First published in 2013 by Lantern Publishing Limited

First edition published in 2009 by Reflect Press (ISBN 978 1 906052 19 5)

Lantern Publishing Limited, The Old Hayloft, Vantage Business Park, Bloxham Road, Banbury OX16 9UX, UK

www.lanternpublishing.com

**British Library Cataloguing in Publication Data**
A catalogue record for this book is available from the British Library

The authors and publisher have made every attempt to ensure the content of this book is up to date and accurate. However, healthcare knowledge and information is changing all the time, as is government legislation, so the reader is advised to double-check any information in this text on drug usage, treatment procedures, the use of equipment, etc. to confirm that it complies with the latest safety recommendations, standards of practice and legislation, as well as local Trust policies and procedures. Students are advised to check with their tutor and/or mentor before carrying out any of the procedures in this textbook.

Typeset by Medlar Publishing Solutions, India
Cover design by Andrew Magee Design Ltd
Printed and bound by 4Edge Ltd, Hockley, Essex, UK
Distributed by NBN International, 10 Thornbury Road, Plymouth, PL6 7PP, UK

# CONTENTS

# PREFACE

The NMC is responsible for setting standards of proficiency that define the overarching principles of being able to practise as a nurse, and must be achieved before students are eligible to join the register. The aim of this handbook is to highlight and address many of the key issues which surround these standards of proficiency and relate them to working knowledge you require in the practice setting.

The handbook has been written primarily for student nurses, return to practice nurses and those who trained overseas, but it is envisaged that students undertaking Further Education access courses and Qualifications and Credit Framework (QCF) courses in health care will also find the information helpful. The content is also relevant for Health Care Assistants and Assistant Practitioners.

The information within the book is relevant to all areas of nursing, and all branches of nursing. It is designed so that you can utilise individual chapters as a quick source of reference, although along with the activities and further reading, it may serve as a starting point for more in-depth study. Where websites are identified, these are only suggested sources of further information and others may be found through general search engines such as www.google.co.uk. Although the emphasis is mainly related to healthcare in England, we do refer to Scotland, Wales and Northern Ireland when appropriate.

*Wendy Benbow and Gill Jordan*
November 2012

# ABOUT THE AUTHORS

Following qualification as a registered nurse in 1969, **Wendy Benbow** worked for two years in genito-urinary surgery and major spinal injuries before moving into community nursing. Over a 14-year period Wendy was involved in a variety of roles that included community nursing, sister, practice work teacher and nurse manager, as well as time seconded for research and co-ordinating pre-registration student placements for the local acute hospital.

After a year out to complete her teaching qualification, Wendy moved into full-time education in 1985. Since then she has been involved in both teaching on and managing a range of pre- and post-registration courses, programme development, regionally funded research and national project development. She is currently working as an associate lecturer for the Open University.

On qualifying as a registered nurse in 1978, **Gill Jordan** completed her Orthopaedic Nursing Certificate and moved to New Zealand where she worked in a large orthopaedic teaching hospital, ultimately as a ward sister of a trauma orthopaedic ward.

On her return to the UK in 1988, Gill moved into nurse education. Since then, she has been involved in a variety of courses and professional development programmes, as both a teacher and programme leader. These have included courses leading to professional registration, Return to Practice, Overseas Nurses Programme, conversion courses and various post-registration undergraduate programmes.

# 01

# NURSE EDUCATION AND MENTORSHIP

This chapter provides an overview of the preparation nurses undertake during their pre-registration programmes, and an insight into the registered nurse's role in supporting students.

| **Learning Outcomes** | • have an outline view of programmes leading to nurse registration; |
| --- | --- |
| On completion of this chapter you should: | • understand the need for mentorship in nursing; |
| | • be able to define the qualities required to be a good mentor. |

## Pre-registration nurse education

### Background

Before the 1990s, nurse education was a traditional 'apprentice'-style training where nurses were based in a school of nursing within the hospital where they carried out their clinical work. There were then two levels of nurse qualification – Registered Nurse (1$^{st}$ level nurse) and Enrolled Nurse (2$^{nd}$ level nurse). Registered Nurses followed a three-year training programme, while Enrolled Nurses took a more practically based two-year training programme. In the 1980s there was a push towards establishing nursing on a more professional footing, and a recognition that nurses were taking on work more traditionally carried out by doctors, with health care assistants undertaking work that had been carried out by registered nurses. This was coupled with the appreciation that there were common elements that underpinned all nursing practice, whichever 'branch' or 'field' of nursing (mental health, learning disability, adult, child health) was studied.

The 1990s saw the advent of 'Project 2000' – a new style of nurse training that transformed pre-registration nurse education at the time and continues to do so. As you know, nurses now study in universities (higher education institutes) and leave their programme not only with a first-level professional nursing qualification (Registered Nurse), but with a higher-educational qualification as well.

## Nurse education today

The Nursing and Midwifery Council (NMC) sets the standards for pre-registration nursing education (Nursing and Midwifery Order, 2001). These are articulated in the document *Standards for Pre-registration Nursing Education* (NMC, 2010). The standards are informed by the Royal College of Nursing (RCN) definition of nursing as "the use of clinical judgement in the provision of care to enable people to improve, maintain or recover health, to cope with health problems, and to achieve the best possible quality of life, whatever their disease or disability, until death" (RCN, 2004, p. 3). They are also informed by the European Tuning project (Tuning, 2009, cited in NMC, 2010), which adopted this definition of the nurse in 2003:

> A professional person achieving a competent standard of practice at first cycle level following successful completion of an approved academic and practical course. The nurse is a safe, caring, and competent decision maker willing to accept personal and professional accountability for his/her actions and continuous learning. The nurse practises within a statutory framework and code of ethics delivering nursing practice (care) that is appropriately based on research, evidence and critical thinking that effectively responds to the needs of individual clients (patients) and diverse populations.
>
> (NMC, 2010, p. 11)

Within the *Standards* (NMC, 2010) the NMC states that its aim is to ensure the public can be confident that all new nurses will:

- deliver high quality essential care to all;

- deliver complex care to service users in their field of practice;

- act to safeguard the public, and be responsible and accountable for safe, person-centred, evidence-based nursing practice;

- act with professionalism and integrity, and work within agreed professional, ethical and legal frameworks and processes to maintain and improve standards;

- practise in a compassionate, respectful way, maintaining dignity and wellbeing and communicating effectively;

- act on their understanding of how people's lifestyles, environments and the location of care delivery influence their health and wellbeing;

- seek out every opportunity to promote health and prevent illness;

- work in partnership with other health and social care professionals and agencies, service users, carers and families ensuring that decisions about care are shared;

- use leadership skills to supervise and manage others and contribute to planning, designing, delivering and improving future services.

(NMC, 2010, p. 5)

The NMC does not produce a national curriculum for nursing education, but the Council does determine the content of programmes. Equally, it does not set specific requirements for the nature or range of practice learning, other than that it must enable the competencies to be acquired. University programmes have to be validated by the NMC, and are subject to regular reviews. In addition to NMC standards, universities also have to comply with standards set by the Quality Assurance Agency (QAA), which are general standards for all courses run within higher education. From 2013, all students entering a pre-registration nursing programme will undertake a degree level course, which reflects the essential and complex care nurses deliver in many different settings (NMC, 2010).

Nurses enrol on a programme for a 'field' of nursing – adult, child, learning disabilities or mental health – and whichever field is studied, 50 per cent of time is spent on theoretical aspects of nursing and 50 per cent in practice areas. This equates to 2300 hours each of practice and theory with progression points at the end of each year, where both theory and practice competencies have to be achieved.

## Competencies for entry to the register

The NMC has to be satisfied that its standards for granting a person a licence to practise are being met as required, and it does this by setting competencies that must be achieved before you are eligible to join the register.

The standards for competence fall into four domains of practice (NMC, 2010, p. 7):

- professional values;

- communication and interpersonal skills;

- nursing practice and decision-making;

- leadership, management and team working.

Pre-registration education programmes must include (NMC, 2010, pp. 73–75):

- theories of nursing and theories of nursing practice;

- research methods and use of evidence;

- professional codes, ethics, law and humanities;

- communication and health care informatics;

- life sciences (including anatomy and physiology);

- pharmacology and medicines management;

- social, health and behavioural sciences;

- principles of national and international health policy, including public health;

- principles of supervision, leadership and management;

- principles of organisational structures, systems and processes;

- causes of common health conditions and the interaction between physical and mental health and illness;

- best practice;

- health care technology;

- essential first aid and incident management.

In addition the following must be included:

- communication, compassion and dignity;

- emotional support;

- equality, diversity, inclusiveness and rights;

- identity, appearance and self-worth;
- autonomy, independence and self-care;
- public health and promoting health and wellbeing;
- maintaining a safe environment;
- eating, drinking, nutrition and hydration;
- comfort and sleep;
- moving and positioning;
- continence promotion and bowel and bladder care;
- skin health and wound management;
- infection prevention and control;
- clinical observation, assessment, critical thinking and decision-making;
- symptom management, such as anxiety, anger, thirst, pain and breathlessness;
- risk management;
- medicines management;
- information management;
- supervising, leading, managing and promoting best practice.

## FURTHER INFORMATION

For information on specific competencies visit www.nmc-uk.org and view the document *Standards for Pre-registration Nursing Education* (2010).

## Practice placements

Practice placements are an essential and integral part of a nurse education programme. They provide unique learning experiences and opportunities for you as a student, but these need to be planned, structured, managed and co-ordinated in order to enable you to develop professional competencies that cannot be readily acquired elsewhere. Stuart (2003) believes that your clinical experience should be much more than just learning what to do and how to do it – it should be about the education of students who will one day be professional peers, colleagues and co-learners. During practice hours you are deemed supernumerary, which means that you are not included in the permanent staff numbers. You are assessed in practice by a mentor via a set of competencies issued by the NMC (a series of standards that you have to achieve both during and at the end of your three-year programme). Although you are supernumerary, you are generally expected to complete the same shift patterns as your mentor, and to gain experience of night working.

The NMC, in reflecting European Union requirements (2005/36/EC), stipulates that your practice experience must include direct contact with healthy and/or sick individuals, and it must enable you to meet all your relevant statutory requirements. All your hours must be verified. The nature of your placements has to be extensive in order to provide learning opportunities that reflect the large range of health care needs experienced by the population, but the timing, length and type of placement will differ between individual universities (www.nursingcourses.org.uk/pre_registration.html).

The RCN (2006) lists sixteen points it believes are important for your learning in an effective practice placement. Placements should help you to:

- meet the statutory and regulatory requirements and, where applicable, European directives;

- achieve the required learning outcomes and competencies according to regulatory body requirements for pre-registration education;

- recognise the diversity of learning opportunities available within health and social care environments;

- work within a wide range of rapidly changing health and social services that recognise the continuing nature of care;

- provide the full range of nursing care to patients;

- demonstrate an appreciation of the unpredictable and dynamic nature of the clinical setting as a learning environment within a multi-professional approach to care;

- feel valued and safe within a culture that recognises the importance of adult learning;

- maintain your supernumerary status;

- work alongside mentors who are appropriately prepared, creating a partnership with them;

- identify appropriate learning opportunities to meet your learning needs, linking general learning objectives to specific experiences within the practice context;

- use time effectively, creating opportunities to enable the application of theory to practice and vice versa;

- apply knowledge gained in the use of experiential, and enquiry- or problem-based learning, within the practice context;

- reflect contemporary thinking within modern health care to evaluate the effectiveness of care provided, and, based on research evidence, continue to develop your competence in both interpersonal and practical skills;

- give an honest, evaluative feedback of your practice experiences to aid the audit process for the practice placement;

- develop skills in information technology to access information within the placement area.

### ACTIVITY 1.1

The RCN published *Helping Students Get the Best from their Practice Placement* in 2006, which is an excellent document – try to get a copy of this and read through it.

The title 'registered nurse' is protected in law and can only be used by someone registered with the NMC. At the end of your training your course director will complete a declaration of good health and good character on your behalf which must be received by the NMC before it can register you. Once registered, you are accountable to the NMC and have to abide by its standards and guidelines, most importantly *The Code: Standards of Conduct, Performance and Ethics for Nurses and Midwives* (2008a).

## Role of the mentor

Many practice-based professions, including nursing, traditionally rely on clinical staff to support, supervise and teach students in practice settings – the underlying rationale being that in working alongside practitioners, students will learn from experts in a safe, supportive and educationally adjusted environment (Benner, 1984).

The form of support afforded to students can be difficult to define. Within nursing the term 'mentor' is generally used to describe a person who supports and assesses student nurses, while the term 'preceptor' is used for a supporter of a post-registration nurse during their first few months after qualifying. The most popular definition of a mentor comes from the document *Preparation for Mentors and Teachers* (English National Board/Department of Health, 2001, p. 6) which states that 'a mentor is a nurse who facilitates learning and supervises and assesses students in the practice setting'. The NMC states that all students on pre-registration nursing education programmes must be supported and assessed by qualified mentors (NMC, 2010).

Mentors are expected to have the skills to enable you to undergo appropriate and valuable learning experiences and to assess your competence. They must have the equivalent of one year's full-time post-registration experience and be on the same part of the register as you are working towards. They must have undertaken specific preparation for the role consisting of a mentorship course accredited by a Higher Education Institution. The content of such a mentorship course must include (NMC, 2008b, p. 10):

- establishing effective working relationships;
- facilitation of learning;
- assessment and accountability;
- evaluation of learning;
- creating an environment for learning;
- context of practice;
- evidence-based practice;
- leadership.

In addition to this NMC standard, there is an expectation and requirement that all registered nurses play a key part in the preparation of students for registration. This is emphasised explicitly in *The Code* (NMC, 2008a, clause 25) which states that registered nurses must be willing to share their skills and experience for the benefit of their colleagues. Equally, the Department of Health (1999) maintains that every practitioner shares the responsibility to support and teach the next generation of nurses, and that it is important that nurses are taught by those with practical and recent experience of nursing.

## Sign-off mentors

The role of the sign-off mentor was introduced in 2006. This is a mentor who has undergone a mentor preparation course and met additional specific criteria, and is responsible (and accountable) for 'signing-off' a student at the end of their training period. This sign-off confirms you have achieved all your competencies, are fit for practice and have the necessary knowledge, skills and competence to take on the role of a registered nurse.

### ACTIVITY 1.2

Take a few minutes to answer the following questions:

- What qualities would you like to see in your mentor?
- Can you think of any obstacles to being effectively mentored?
- What are the benefits to you as a student of having a mentor?

The RCN (2007, p. 5) states that mentors are required to offer you support and guidance, and to help you make sense of your practice through:

- the application of theory;
- assessing, evaluating and giving constructive feedback;
- facilitating reflection on practice, performance and experiences.

In addition a mentor should:

- be a positive role model;
- be knowledgeable and skilled;
- help you develop skills and confidence;
- promote a professional relationship with you;
- provide you with the appropriate level of supervision;
- assist with planned learning experiences;
- offer honest and constructive feedback.

However, it is not only your mentor who has responsibilities to you; you also have a responsibility (RCN, 2006) to:

- be proactive in seeking out experiences for your level of practice and competence with the support of your mentor;

- demonstrate a willingness to work as part of the team in the delivery of safe patient care;

- learn to express your needs and adopt a questioning, reflective approach to your learning within the multidisciplinary team;

- use your mentor for guidance and support to enable you to achieve your learning outcomes and satisfactorily complete your practice assessments;

- seek help from appropriate clinical managers or link lecturers if the mentor relationship is not working, to enable the achievement of the learning outcomes;

- ensure that clinical skills required at each stage in the programme are attempted under the supervision of a skilled practitioner, with comments provided by both you and your mentor;

- utilise learning opportunities outside the practice placements and, where possible, work with specialist practitioners;

- identify the role of professionals within other contexts of the organisation or community, for example, in X-ray, pharmacy and outpatients;

- give and receive constructive feedback;

- reflect on your progress to increase self-awareness, confidence and competence.

You must also (RCN, 2007):

- read your higher education institution's (HEI's) charter and student handbooks;

- familiarise yourself with handbooks related to your specific programme (these will include assessment of practice documentation);

- recognise the purpose of your placement experience and ensure you are clear about the expectations of the placement provider;

- ensure you have some theoretical knowledge relating to the placement;

- contact your placement and mentor prior to starting;

- highlight any support needs to your mentor;

- act professionally with regard to punctuality, attitude and image, and dress according to uniform policy;

- maintain confidentiality;

- maintain effective communication with patients, mentors and link personnel from both the placement and HEI;

- adhere to the NMC *Guidance on Professional Conduct for Nursing and Midwifery Students* (2011).

As previously stated, one of the major roles of the mentor is to assess you on your clinical practice. All mentors can assess specific competencies and confirm their achievement, but only sign-off mentors can confirm overall achievement of proficiency and therefore fitness for entry to the register. Your consistency of performance is measured via continuous assessment which is, for the most part, by your mentor directly observing the care that you deliver. This is recorded within your 'Ongoing Achievement of Practice Record' which it is your responsibility to take from placement to placement.

---

**FURTHER INFORMATION**

Along with *Helping Students get the Best from their Practice Placement* (RCN, 2006) the RCN also publishes a booklet *Guidance for Mentors of Nursing Students and Midwifery* (RCN, 2007), which you may find helpful.

---

# Preceptorship

There is a general acknowledgement that all professions need a period of transition following qualification for professional registration, and this of course includes nursing. The Department of Health (2010) published a Preceptorship Framework stating that all newly registered practitioners (nurses, midwives and allied health professionals) should undergo a period of preceptorship, defining this as:

> a period of structured transition for the newly registered practitioner
> during which he or she will be supported by a preceptor, to develop
> their confidence as an autonomous professional, refine skills, values
> and behaviours and to continue on their journey of life-long learning.
> (Department of Health, 2010, p. 11)

The precise length of preceptorship will vary according to individual need and local circumstances, but the Department of Health believes that six to twelve months is a suitable time. It acknowledges that every time a newly registered practitioner works alongside more experienced professional colleagues, they can learn from them and be guided by them in many ways. Formal preceptorship, however, means that the newly registered nurse is allocated a named individual, working in the same area of practice, who is on hand to guide, help, advise and support. The NMC states (2005, p. 1) that: "this doesn't mean that they accompany the newly registered nurse everywhere they go and constantly look over their shoulder, but it does mean they can be called if help is needed with a procedure or a situation not encountered before; or if they simply feel that they need support and guidance".

Preceptors, like mentors, must be first-level registered nurses who have had at least twelve months' experience as a registered nurse and understand the concept of preceptorship. There are no formal qualifications to be a preceptor, but preceptors must (NMC, 2006, p. 1):

- know about the newly registered nurse's training and experience and be able to identify learning needs;

- help the newly registered nurse apply knowledge to practice;

- be able to act as a resource to facilitate the newly qualified nurse's professional development.

The content of a preceptorship programme is prescribed as including the following (Department of Health, 2010):

- team working;

- decision-making;

- confidence in applying evidence-based practice;

- development of confidence and self-awareness;

- implementation of codes of professional values;

- increase of knowledge and clinical skills;

- integrating prior learning into practice;

- understanding policies and procedures;

- reflection and receiving feedback;

- development of an outcome-based approach to continuing professional development;

- advocacy;

- interpersonal skills;

- management of risk and not being risk averse;

- equality and diversity;

- negotiation and conflict resolution;

- leadership and management development.

Most NHS Trusts run preceptorship courses within their organisations. Some courses are affiliated to universities and nurses can gain academic credit for successfully completing the scheme of study.

An excellent website with an on-line preceptorship programme can be found at: www.flyingstartengland.nhs.uk (or www.flyingstart.scot.nhs.uk for those based in Scotland).

## Chapter summary

- The NMC sets the standards for pre-registration education – from 2013 all students entering a pre-registration course will study at degree level.

- Students can study for inclusion on the NMC Register in the branches of adult, child or mental health, or learning disability.

- All courses leading to registration are 50 per cent practice and 50 per cent theory.

- All students have to achieve NMC practice competencies to enable them to register, and are allocated a mentor who assesses them in their clinical placements.

- All newly qualified nurses undertake a period of preceptorship on qualifying, organised by their employer.

# References

Benner, P. (1984) *From Novice to Expert.* California: Addison-Wesley.

Department of Health (1999) *Making a Difference: Strengthening the Nursing, Midwifery and Health Visiting Contribution to Health and Healthcare,* London: HMSO.

Department of Health (2010) *Preceptorship Framework for Newly Registered Nurses, Midwives and Allied Health Professionals.* London: Department of Health.

English National Board/Department of Health (2001) *Preparation of Mentors and Teachers – A New Framework Guidance.* London: ENB/Department of Health.

Nursing and Midwifery Council (2005) *Supporting Nurses and Midwives through Lifelong Learning.* London: NMC.

Nursing and Midwifery Council (2006) *Preceptorship Guidelines,* 21/2006. London: NMC.

Nursing and Midwifery Council (2008a) *The Code: Standards of Conduct, Performance and Ethics for Nurses and Midwives,* London: NMC.

Nursing and Midwifery Council (2008b) *Standards to Support Learning and Assessment in Practice.* London: NMC.

Nursing and Midwifery Council (2010) *Standards for Pre-registration Nursing Education.* London: NMC.

Nursing and Midwifery Council (2011) *Guidance on Professional Conduct for Nursing and Midwifery Students.* London: NMC.

Nursing and Midwifery Order (2001) www.nmc-uk.org/About-us/legislation/the-order/ (accessed 19 November 2012)

Royal College of Nursing (2004) *The Future Nurse: The RCN Vision.* London: RCN.

Royal College of Nursing (2006) *Helping Students get the Best from their Practice Placement.* London: RCN.

Royal College of Nursing (2007) *Guidance for Mentors of Nursing Students and Midwives.* London: RCN.

Stuart, C. (2003) *Assessment, Supervision and Support in Clinical Practice.* London: Churchill Livingstone.

www.nmc-uk.org (accessed 19 November 2012)

www.learning-styles-online.com (accessed 19 November 2012)

www.nursingcourses.org.uk/pre_registration.html (accessed 10 December 2012)

# 02
# COMMUNICATION

**The aim of this chapter is to introduce briefly the concept of communication in the context of health care delivery.**

| **Learning Outcomes** | • understand the definitions and the process of communication; |
|---|---|
| On completion of this chapter you should: | • be able to identify and overcome the barriers that may prevent effective communication taking place; |
| | • understand the skills required for effective and active listening; |
| | • have explored the concept of emotional quotient / intelligence. |

## Introduction

As a student nurse you will be required to develop and maintain a high level of intra- and interpersonal communication. In fact it is probably one of the most important skills you will need, wherever your area of practice might be, because you must be able to communicate effectively to provide competent nursing care. Despite this importance it is well recognised that many practitioners do not always communicate with others as well as they should.

## Communication defined

A considerable number of definitions of communication can be found in the literature; here are just a few.

• The process by which we understand others and in turn endeavour to be understood by them (Burnard, 1997).

- A two-way process of reaching mutual understanding, in which participants not only exchange information but also create and share meaning (www.businessdictionary.com).

- A complex process of sending and receiving verbal and non-verbal messages that allows for an exchange of information, feelings, needs and preferences (www1.villanova.edu).

- In nursing, communication is a sharing of health-related information between a patient and a nurse, with both participants as sources and receivers. The information may be verbal or non-verbal, written or spoken, personal or impersonal, issue-specific or even relationship-orientated (Sheldon, 2004, p4).

## The communication process

One way of beginning to explain how communication occurs is the baseline process model of communication (see *Figure 2.1*). Based on the work of Shannon and Weaver (1949) this model is still one of the most widely used as a starting point to understand the process of communication.

The communication process is made up of four key components, as shown in *Figure 2.1*.

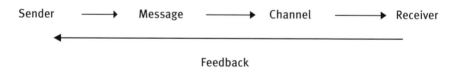

*Figure 2.1 – A process model of communication*

### The sender (transmitter)

The sender is an individual, group or organisation that initiates the communication. All communication begins with the sender and the source is initially responsible for the success of the message. The first step for the sender involves the encoding process.

### The message

In order to convey meaning the sender must translate (encode) information into a message in the form of symbols that represent ideas, concepts, etc. These symbols can take numerous forms such as languages, words or gestures. It is clearly important for the sender to use symbols that are familiar to and appropriate for the intended receiver.

## The channel

The channel is the means by which the sender conveys the message. Channels or types of communication generally come under the main headings:

- verbal;
- non-verbal;
- tactile;
- written.

## The receiver

After the appropriate channel or channels have been selected, the message enters the decoding stage of the communication process. Decoding is conducted by the receiver. Once the message is received, the stimulus is sent to the brain for interpreting in order to assign some type of meaning. The receiver translates the message into their own set of experiences in order to make the symbols meaningful. All interpretations by the receiver are influenced by their experiences, attitudes, knowledge, skills, perceptions and culture (as with the sender's encoding) (Sherman, 1994; Reynolds, 1997; Foulger, 2004).

Although, according to this model, communication is seemingly a simple activity, in essence it is not. It is a complex process in which many other factors need to be considered for effective communication to take place.

# Interpersonal skills

Put simply, interpersonal skills are the skills we use to interact or deal with others.

Allender and Spradley (2005) suggest that in nursing there are three particular types of interpersonal skills that build on sending and receiving skills, and these are:

- respect;
- rapport;
- trust.

## Respect

According to Peate (2006, p. 130) respect relates to the ability of a nurse to demonstrate a sincere interest in the patient and his or her needs. Expressing a genuine wish to understand, showing kindness and patience, and being concerned for any fears or discomfort the patient may have are all ways of demonstrating respect to the patient and their family.

## Rapport

Rapport links to showing respect and is about sympathetic and harmonious relationships, especially ones of emotional affinity and mutual trust.

## Trust

Trust is about integrity and having faith and confidence in another person. In nursing, Allender and Spradley (2005) suggest that trust is developed by providing an open, honest and patient-focused approach.

## Empathy

A further interpersonal skill that is important to mention here is empathy. Definitions of empathy are many but essentially it is about the attempt to understand and share, in a non-judgemental way, the feelings, experiences and concerns of others. Empathy for the most part is a learnt skill or attitude and although it is unlikely that a person who develops such a skill could ever know exactly what another person actually feels, it is important that the nurse should learn to make the attempt to do so. Empathising with a patient, a carer, etc., can only enhance the ability to communicate effectively (www.scips.worc.ac.uk).

### ACTIVITY 2.1

Take a few minutes to reflect back on one or two experiences of being involved in caring for someone where you have utilised the four interpersonal skills identified above.

# Emotional intelligence

A relatively recent behavioural model linked to communication and interpersonal skills is that of Emotional Intelligence (EI). Emotional intelligence describes an ability to perceive, assess and manage one's own emotions and those of others ([www.psychology.about.com](www.psychology.about.com)).

The EI concept suggests that IQ (intelligence quotient), the traditional measure of intelligence, is too limiting as it ignores essential behavioural and character elements. EI encompasses the wider areas of intelligence that dictate and contribute to how successful an individual is. An example often used is that of a person who can be academically brilliant and yet socially and interpersonally inept; we know that despite their possessing a high IQ rating, success does not automatically follow.

Essentially EI has two main aspects, namely:

- understanding yourself;
- understanding others and their feelings.

Within these aspects there are four key dimensions:

- **Self-awareness** – knowing one's internal states, preferences, goals, intentions, etc.
- **Social awareness** – awareness of the feelings, needs and concerns of others.
- **Self-management** – managing one's internal states, impulses and resources to facilitate reaching goals.
- **Social skills** – adeptness at inducing desirable responses in others.

Extensive research on the subject appears to suggest that the process and outcomes of EI development contain many elements known to reduce stress for individuals and organisations, by decreasing conflict and improving relationships and understanding. Also, those who exhibit a high degree of EI tend to be more fulfilled and productive than others in every area of their lives: personal, professional, and family (Titimae, 2006; Russell, 2007; [www.businessballs.com](www.businessballs.com)).

## ACTIVITY 2.2

There is a considerable amount of information on the internet with regard to emotional intelligence. This includes many sites that provide an opportunity to measure your own level of EI. As a starting point just use a general search engine such as Google.

# Non-verbal interaction

Verbal and non-verbal skills are closely interrelated and thus non-verbal interaction in health care is also extremely important. Faulkner (1997, p. 76) suggests that, generally, if concurrent verbal and non-verbal messages do not match, then the non-verbal message is the one more likely to be believed.

Non-verbal interaction includes the following:

- **Gesture** – e.g. with hands, arms, head. The gestures people use convey meanings; for example, arms firmly crossed and head turned away can give a negative message to the receiver.

- **Posture** – e.g. sit, stand, slouch. The way that we stand or sit gives information about how we are feeling; for example, a nurse sitting slumped in a chair can also give a negative message.

- **Facial expressions** – our faces can show many of our feelings. For example, a frown or a smile shows a very clear message depending on how and when it is used.

- **Eye contact** – maintaining appropriate eye contact when speaking with others helps positive communication. Avoiding eye contact may suggest that you do not really want to communicate, or that you may be telling a lie. Although eye contact for several seconds is good, you should also be aware that staring or excessive eye contact may make a person feel uncomfortable.

- **Proximity** – most people feel uncomfortable when somebody stands or sits either too close or too far away from them. When this situation happens, it can make communication more difficult.

There is no doubt that when you focus on combining verbal and non-verbal messages in the most effective way possible you should significantly improve your overall communication skills.

---

### ACTIVITY 2.3

The next time you interact with a patient, carer, etc. stop and think about your non-verbal communication – what message/s do you think you are conveying to the receiver of your message?

# Barriers to effective communication

Unfortunately there are many ways in which the message being transmitted in the communication process either never reaches the receiver, or fails to be understood or is misinterpreted by the receiver. Such barriers to effective communication include the following:

- Non-verbal:

    - negative messages from body language.

- Linguistic:

    - speaking too quickly or too slowly;

    - too much or too little information given at one time;

    - language differences;

    - regional or national accents;

    - use of technical jargon;

    - restricted or elaborate code of speech;

    - level of voice;

    - tone of voice.

- Cultural:

    - different values, social norms, rules and rituals (this relates to both verbal and non-verbal communication), and can include social class, perceptions and prejudices.

- Social:

    - background and education;

    - status of the sender – communication is easier if perceived power differential is low.

- Individual/personal:

    - emotional state of the receiver;

    - sensory deficits;

    - poor cognitive skills;

- fatigue;

- mistrust;

- past experiences;

- need to know – is the information being received important to the receiver or not?

- External / structural

  - appropriate place for communication (e.g. is privacy required?);

  - noise;

  - distractions.

---

**ACTIVITY 2.4**

Note down a few key points that you think may help overcome some of the barriers to effective communication listed above.

---

## Overcoming communication barriers

The following are a few points to consider when communicating with service users and their families:

- Select the best location – communicate somewhere that will encourage effective communication.

- Being positive and supportive rather than negative and defensive helps make communication more effective.

- Ensure the best channel for communication has been chosen.

- Be respectful and empathise if appropriate.

- Always be culturally and socially aware with regard to those with whom you are communicating.

- Ensure communication is clear, concise, concrete, correct and courteous.

- Use repetition – repeating messages using different examples or channels can sometimes help the receiver to understand the message being sent.

- Check written communication for spelling errors and ensure the sentences are clear, concise and not ambiguous.

- Develop good listening skills.

(Burnard, 1997; Adams, 2007; Peate, 2006; www.witold.me.uk; www.scribd.com)

## Listening skills

In health care listening is an integral and important part of the communication process. However, it can also be one of the most challenging skills for the nurse to develop. The following can be barriers to effective listening.

- Verbal activities, e.g.:

  - interrupting;

  - asking questions at inappropriate times;

  - preoccupation with other issues;

  - noise;

  - individual bias and prejudices;

  - hearing only what you want to hear;

  - trying to work out what the speaker means rather than listening to what is actually being said.

- Non-verbal activities, e.g.:

  - avoiding eye contact;

  - bored expression, yawning;

  - fiddling and fidgeting;

  - checking watches;

  - tidying papers, etc;

  - perceived time restriction;

  - inattention generally.

Unfortunately, some of the above activities happen far too frequently in the busy area of health care practice.

## Good listening skills

Good listening skills are not just about being silent and passively receiving the thoughts and feelings of others. To be an effective listener, you need to respond with verbal and non-verbal cues which communicate to the speaker that you are listening to what they are saying. Good listening skills include:

- Give the speaker your undivided attention and look at the speaker directly (not at what else is going on around you).

- Make sure your mind is focused. If you feel your mind wandering, change the position of your body and try to concentrate on the speaker's words.

- Listen for main ideas. Pay special attention to statements that begin with phrases such as 'My point is...' or 'The thing to remember is...'. Also 'listen' to the speaker's non-verbal cues.

- Show you are listening – use body language to convey your attention. For example, nod occasionally, smile and use facial expressions, ensure your posture is open and welcoming.

- Don't interrupt; let the speaker finish before you begin to talk and let yourself finish listening before you begin to speak. Wait for the right opportunity to ask questions.

- If you are not sure you understand what the speaker has said, you need to check with them to ensure your understanding is correct. This may be achieved by repeating their words (for example, the last few words of the sentence) or by reflecting back in your own words (paraphrasing) what the speaker has said.

- Keep an open and receptive mind to people and their thoughts.

- Be respectful and courteous at all times.

Remember that listening takes time or, more accurately, that you have to take time to listen (Peate, 2006; www.mindtools.com; www.infoplease.com).

### FURTHER READING

Burnard, P. and Gill, P. (2008) *Culture, Communication and Nursing: A Multicultural Guide* – explores in more depth the wider issues associated with culture and communication.

Donnelly, E. and Neville, L. (2008) *Health and Social Care Knowledge and Skills: Communication and Interpersonal Skills* – provides an opportunity to further explore the theory that underpins communication studies and also self-assess your own communication and interpersonal skills.

## Chapter summary

- The communication process is made up of four key components, i.e. the sender, a message, a channel and the receiver.

- Interpersonal skills are the skills we use to interact or deal with others.

- Emotional intelligence is a behavioural model linked to communication and interpersonal skills and describes the ability to perceive, access and manage one's own emotions and those of others.

- Verbal and non-verbal interaction and skills are closely related and both are extremely important in health care.

- Barriers to effective communication are numerous, therefore an understanding of what they might be and how they might be overcome is critical.

- Listening is an integral part of the communication process. To be an effective listener you need to respond with verbal and non-verbal cues which communicate to the speaker that you are listening.

## References

Adams, R. (ed.) (2007) *Foundations in Health and Social Care*. Hampshire: Palgrave Macmillan.

Allender, J.A., and Spradley, W. (2005) *Community Health Nursing: Promoting and Protecting the Public's Health* (6th edition). Philadelphia: Lippincott.

Burnard, P. (1997) *Effective Communication Skills For Health Professionals* (2nd edition). London: Chapman Hall.

Faulkner, A. (1997) *Effective Interaction with Patients*. Edinburgh: Churchill Livingstone.

Foulger, D. (2004) *Models of the Communication Process.* Available from davis.foulger.info/research/unifiedModelOfCommunication.htm (accessed 7 January 2013)

Peate, I. (2006) *Becoming a Nurse in the 21st Century*. Chichester: Wiley.

Reynolds, K. (1997) *What is the Transmission of Interpersonal Communication and what is wrong with it?* Available from www.aber.ac.uk/media/Students/kjr9601.html (accessed 7 January 2013)

Russell, J. (2007) *How's your Emotional Intelligence? Competencies for Enhancing your Effectiveness by Building Healthy and Productive Relationships at Work.* Available from www.russellconsultinginc.com/docs/pdf/bmf_ei_ppt_2007.pdf (accessed 20 November 2012)

Shannon, C.E. and Weaver, W. (1949) *A Mathematical Model of Communication*. Urbana: University of Illinois Press.

Sheldon, L.K. (2004) *Communication for Nurses: Talking with Patients.* Available from http://nursing.flinders.edu.au/students/studyaids/clinicalcommunication/page.php?id = 20 (accessed 20 November 2012)

Sherman, K.M. (1994) *Communication and Image in Nursing*. Delmar: New York.

Titimae, M.A. (2006) *Emotional Intelligence, Management Concept: A Contributing Factor for Effective Service Delivery.* Available from www.mnre.gov.ws/documents/forum/2006/6-mulipola.pdf (accessed 7 January 2013)

www.businessballs.com/eq.htm (accessed 20 November 2012)

www.witold.me.uk/communication.htm (accessed 20 November 2012)

www.scribd.com/doc/10868863/Barriers-to-Communication (accessed 20 November 2012)

www.businessdictionary.com (accessed 20 November 2012)

http://www.scips.worc.ac.uk/subjects_and_challenges/nursing/nursing_empathy.html (accessed 20 November 2012)

http://psychology.about.com/od/personalitydevelopment/a/
emotionalintell.htm (accessed 20 November 2012)

www.mindtools.com/CommSkll/ActiveListening.htm (accessed
20 November 2012)

www.infoplease.com/homework/listeningskills1.html (accessed
20 November 2012)

www06.homepage.villanova.edu/elizabeth.bruderle/1103/communication.htm
(accessed 20 November 2012)

# 03
## LEGAL AND PROFESSIONAL ISSUES

> The aim of this chapter is to make you aware of the legal and professional issues surrounding nursing.
>
> | **Learning Outcomes** | • demonstrate an awareness of the legal framework within which care is provided; |
> |---|---|
> | On completion of this chapter you should be able to: | • discuss the legal responsibilities of nurses when caring for patients or clients; |
> | | • define the term 'accountability' in relation to *The Code: Standards of Conduct, Performance and Ethics* (NMC, 2008a) and other guidelines issued by the Nursing and Midwifery Council. |

You may not feel that all the considerations discussed in this chapter apply to you as you are not yet a Nursing and Midwifery Council (NMC) registrant. However, as a citizen or resident of the United Kingdom (UK) the legal aspects do apply (under both criminal and civil law). In addition you are advised to look on the NMC regulations as a guide for best practice. Any employment regulation may affect you when undertaking clinical practice and you should also be aware of any charters, guidelines, policies, etc. that your university or college and/or placement organisation asks you to respect.

## Accountability

'To be accountable is literally to be liable to be called upon to give an account of what one has done or not done' (Banks, 2004, p. 150). The importance of accountability in professional life is not new, but there is an increasing focus on issues around nursing accountability and nurses, both registered and in preparation for registration, must be aware of its implications.

Accountability is often defined as responsibility, but there is a difference between the two. Responsibility is concerned with answering for what you do, whereas accountability is being answerable for the 'consequences' of what you do. The most important factor in accountability is that it is 'personal' and no other registered nurse can be accountable for another. The NMC (2008a, p. 1) states this very clearly in *The Code: Standards of Conduct, Performance and Ethics for Nurses and Midwives* (referred to as *The Code* from here on):

> 'As a professional, you are personally accountable for actions and omissions in your practice, and must always be able to justify your decisions.
>
> You must always act lawfully, whether those laws relate to your professional practice or personal life.'

Before registration you are not *professionally* accountable in the way that you will be after registering with the NMC. However, the NMC clearly states that as a student you must conduct yourself professionally at all times in order to justify the trust the public places in the professions (NMC, 2011a).

Castledine (1991) offers a further definition of accountability which encompasses the whole ethos of how accountability in nursing should be viewed. He states that accountability is:

> 'that special phenomena [sic] related to nursing practice which nurses are entrusted with, are answerable for, take the credit and the blame for, and can be judged within legal and moral boundaries'.
>
> Castledine (1991, p. 28).

This chapter explores those legal boundaries.

## Arenas of accountability

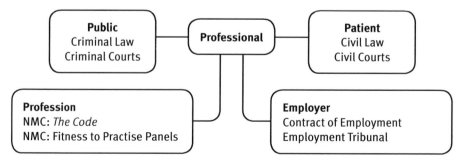

Figure 3.1 – Arenas of accountability (adapted from Dimond, 2011)

As you can see from *Figure 3.1*, Dimond (2011), a barrister who has a great interest in professional accountability and patients' rights, believes there are four arenas of accountability which nurses must consider.

## Criminal law and the courts

In criminal law, a crime is committed against the state either when an act is performed that the law forbids, or when an act is omitted that the law requires. For a conviction it must be proved that a person intended to commit the crime, or was reckless in doing the criminal act. More serious cases include murder, manslaughter and rape (all of which nurses have been found guilty of) and are heard in a Crown Court before a judge and jury. Lesser cases (such as driving offences) are heard in a magistrates' court. The outcome of prosecution is a custodial sentence or a fine, or both.

## Civil law and the courts

This part of the law involves the rights and duties individuals have towards each other. Legal action can be taken by a private individual against another individual or an organisation. This is the main area which affects nurses and which lawyers refer to as the law of torts. The outcomes from these cases usually involve awards of compensation (for damages) or orders (injunctions) to stop an individual acting unlawfully. The NMC recognises that this is an area where nurses are increasingly being involved and since 2004 has included a section in *The Code* in which it recommends that registered nurses have professional indemnity insurance – 'in the event of claims of professional negligence' (NMC, 2008a, clause 62).

### Duty of care (negligence)

An action for negligence is a civil action, and results from a breach of duty of care. A nurse may be held legally liable if it can be shown either that they have failed to exercise the skills properly expected of them, or that they have undertaken tasks that they are not competent to perform (Dimond, 2011).

For negligence to be proved the following conditions must be satisfied:
1. A duty of care is owed by the defendant (nurse) to the claimant (patient) i.e. the nurse / patient relationship (duty);
2. There is a breach in the standard of care owed (breach);
3. This breach has caused reasonably foreseeable harm (causation);
4. This breach has caused harm, either by action or omission.

Some criminal cases may also have a civil action brought if any harm has been caused by 'action or omission'.

---

**ACTIVITY 3.1**

- Think of a circumstance where a nurse might be held criminally liable (i.e. a criminal act that a nurse might commit).
- Think of circumstances in clinical practice where a nurse might be judged negligent (i.e. perform an act that could be referred to a civil court).

---

### Accountability to the employer

All those in a nursing role are accountable to their employer. There is an implied term in every contract of employment that the employee will obey the reasonable instructions of the employer (i.e. follow any policies, procedures, standards, etc.), and that any employee who breaches their contract may be subject to disciplinary action. Even though, as a student nurse, you are not 'employed' by a placement organisation as such, you are still bound by their 'instructions', and any deviation from these could lead to disciplinary action by your university and/or your placement provider. You must therefore be familiar with the policies, procedures, etc. of your placement provider, as you could be called to account by your university or by the law.

#### Vicarious liability

Employers are liable for any actions committed by their employees (for example nurses) during the scope of their employment. The employer (for example, an NHS Trust or a care home) cannot shirk this liability by saying it provides competent, trained staff – it will always be primarily responsible for any negligence to patients by their staff (Dimond, 2011).

However, this does not remove any legal responsibility / accountability from the nurse. If a patient takes a civil action against a hospital (for example, for damages caused by one of its employees), and the hospital is found directly liable by the civil courts, the hospital as the employer could in turn take legal action against the employee. This usually happens when a hospital (an employer) has to pay compensation to a patient as a result of an employee's negligence, and tries to recoup their money from the employee. As this falls in the arena of civil law, which applies to all citizens and residents of the UK, this could affect you as a student nurse.

# The Nursing and Midwifery Council

The core function of the NMC is to establish standards of education, training, conduct and performance for nursing and midwifery and to ensure those standards are maintained, thereby safeguarding the health and wellbeing of the public. The powers of the NMC are set out in the Nursing and Midwifery Order 2001. Although you are a student nurse, you are already affected by the role of the NMC as it sets the standards of education and training you are undertaking. The NMC determines the level of entry and content of pre-registration nursing programmes, and universities have to have validation from the NMC to run such programmes. Programmes are also monitored and reviewed by the NMC on a regular basis.

The NMC's key tasks are to:

• safeguard the health and wellbeing of the public;

• set standards of education, training and conduct so that nurses and midwives can deliver high quality healthcare consistently throughout their careers;

• ensure nurses and midwives keep their skills and knowledge up to date and uphold professional standards;

• have clear and transparent processes to investigate nurses and midwives who fall short of standards.

(NMC, 2011a, p. i)

All nurses working in a registered nurse capacity must be registered with the NMC. When you have successfully completed your nursing programme your university will notify the NMC that you have met the required standards and that you are eligible for entry on the register. Your course director will also complete a Declaration of Good Health and Good Character on your behalf, which must be received by the NMC before registration can take place.

## What constitutes good health and good character?

Good health and good character are fundamental to fitness to practise as a nurse.

**Good health** means that you must be capable of safe and effective practice without supervision. It does not mean the absence of any disability or health condition. Many disabled people and those with health conditions are able to practise, with or without adjustments to support their practice.

Long-term conditions such as epilepsy, diabetes or depression can be well managed and would not be incompatible with registration. Equally, temporary health conditions do not necessarily mean a person is not fit to practise. For example, having a broken leg may mean a person is not fit to work for a period of time. It does not mean they are not fit to practise as they can reasonably expect to recover fully and return to work.

**Good character** is important as nurses and midwives must be honest and trustworthy. Your good character is based on your conduct, behaviour and attitude. It covers examples such as someone who knowingly practises as a nurse before they are on the register, or someone who signs a student off from an educational programme while being aware of poor behaviour.

It also includes any convictions and cautions that are not considered compatible with professional registration and that might bring the profession into disrepute. Your character must be sufficiently good for you to be capable of safe and effective practice without supervision (NMC, 2011a).

---

**ACTIVITY 3.2**

Visit the NMC website (www.nmc-uk.org/Students/Good-Health-and-Good-Character-for-students-nurses-and-midwives) and read the information posted there.

---

## Guidance on professional conduct for nursing and midwifery students

The NMC acknowledges that as a student you will come into close contact with patients, by observing care being given, by helping to provide care and, towards the end of your course, through full participation in providing care. As a student nurse you are bound by the NMC *Guidance on professional conduct for nursing and midwifery students* (2011a) which states you must conduct yourself professionally at all times 'in order to justify the trust the public place in our professions' (NMC, 2011a, p. 3).

This guidance clearly states the attitude and behaviour expected of you, not just in the clinical setting, but also in your university or college. It outlines the role of the NMC and describes its vision, mission and values in its introduction, and it links the expectations of student conduct with the NMC Code for registered nurses which you will be required to adhere to once you qualify (NMC, 2011a).

Along with guidance on many aspects of your clinical role the NMC emphasises that as a student you must 'recognise and stay within the limits of your competence' and 'work only under the supervision and support of a qualified professional and ask for help from your mentor or tutor when you need it' (NMC, 2011a, p. 15). In addition it states the conduct expected of you as a university student:

- to take responsibility for your own learning;

- to follow the policy on attendance as set out by your university and clinical placement provider;

- to follow the policy on submission of coursework and completion of clinical assessments as set out by your university and clinical placement provider;

- to reflect on and respond constructively to feedback you are given;

- to endeavour to provide care based on the best available evidence or best practice;

- not to plagiarise or falsify coursework or clinical assessments.

(NMC, 2011a, pp. 16–17)

## ACTIVITY 3.3

Visit the NMC website (www.nmc-uk.org) and download and read *Guidance on Professional Conduct for Nursing and Midwifery Students* (2011). This sets out your responsibilities as a student.

## *The Code: Standards of Conduct, Performance and Ethics for Nurses and Midwives* (2008a)

Once registered, you must be aware of the professional accountability you will automatically assume. The NMC stresses the need for all registered nurses to be personally accountable for their practice by issuing them with

*The Code: Standards of Conduct, Performance and Ethics for Nurses and Midwives* (NMC, 2008a). Although this document is not part of law, the functions of the NMC include a requirement to establish and improve standards of professional conduct (Health Act, 1999; Nursing and Midwifery Order, 2001), and they do this by issuing *The Code* and a requirement for all registered nurses to abide by it. Breaching *The Code* is in effect a breach of registration and may lead to the removal of the nurse's name from the register:

> Failure to comply with this Code of Conduct may bring your fitness to practise into question and endanger your registration.
>
> (NMC, 2008a, p. 1)

Paramount in *The Code* is the requirement for registered nurses to have 'the knowledge and skills for safe and effective practice' (NMC, 2008a, clause 38). In line with this the NMC warns that careful consideration must be made of professional accountability if nurses are asked to work in an area for which they are not adequately prepared – being open about their limitations is not a sign of weakness but rather a key indicator of mature and caring practice (Richards and Edwards, 2008). *The Code* (NMC, 2008a, clauses 39 and 41) endorses this by stating:

> You must recognize and work within the limits of your competence.
>
> You must take part in appropriate learning and practice activities that maintain and develop your competence and performance.

*The Code* is divided into four sections with a number of subsections. The whole code is prefaced with the words (NMC, 2008a, p. 1):

> The people in your care must be able to trust you with their health and wellbeing. To justify that trust, you must...

And then indicates the four main sections:

- make the care of people your first concern, treating them as individuals and respecting their dignity;

- work with others to protect and promote the health and wellbeing of those in your care, their families and carers, and the wider community;

- provide a high standard of practice and care at all times;

- be open and honest, act with integrity and uphold the reputation of your profession.

The introduction continues:

> As a professional, you are personally accountable for actions and omissions in your practice and must always be able to justify your decisions.
>
> You must always act lawfully, whether those laws relate to your professional practice or personal life.

This code of conduct should be considered together with the Nursing and Midwifery Council's rules, standards, guidance and advice available from www.nmc-uk.org.

# Delegation

Although *The Code* emphasises that all registered nurses are personally accountable for their practice, there may be some instances where nurses may be delegated tasks, or indeed delegate tasks themselves.

The NMC has a section in *The Code* (NMC, 2008a, clauses 29–31) outlining the considerations nurses must take before delegating:

- you must establish that anyone you delegate to is able to carry out your instructions;

- you must confirm that the outcome of any delegated task meets the required standards;

- you must make sure that everyone you are responsible for is supervised and supported.

This last clause could affect you if you believe that a registered nurse has delegated you a task and is not supporting or supervising you. As mentioned above, the NMC states that, as a student, you must: 'recognise and stay within the limits of your competence' and 'work only under the supervision and support of a qualified professional and ask for help from your mentor or tutor when you need it' (NMC, 2011a, p. 1).

Peate (2006) reminds registered nurses of the legal perspective of delegation, and believes that when delegating a task the following must be borne in mind:

- when working as a team member you are personally accountable for your own actions or omissions – there is no such concept as team negligence. If harm occurs, you are individually accountable;

## ACTIVITY 3.4

Obtain a copy of *The Code* from the NMC website (www.nmc-uk.org). Read it and then read the following article and identify the sections of *The Code* you think this nurse breached – the answers are in the conclusion at the end of the activity.

(Reproduced with permission from *British Journal of Nursing*)

### Staff nurse who failed to provide adequate nursing care for patients

*British Journal of Nursing*, 2004, Vol. 13, No 7:389 Professional Misconduct Series

In the following case a senior nurse called Jo deliberately ignored certain aspects of care while on night duty because she felt that it was not her responsibility to carry out certain tasks or to check that they had been done.

Jo worked on nights for a large inner-city hospital trust and had been doing so for over 10 years. When working on the general medical / surgical wards she was often heard to say derogatory remarks about some of the patients or core nursing tasks she was expected to do. For example, she saw it as a junior nursing role to go round and attend to patients' pressure needs. She felt her expertise lay in giving out drugs, managing intravenous infusion lines and doing certain nursing procedures.

On the particular ward where she was working two patients requested pain relief. Jo did not bother to go and see the patients, but instructed two healthcare assistants who were on duty with her to give each of the patients two paracetamol tablets. The healthcare assistants gave the medication to the patients as directed, but at no time did Jo attempt to check what they had given or to clarify with the patients how they were feeling. The situation continued for several shifts. Any patient who required additional pain relief was referred by the healthcare assistants to Jo, who told them to give paracetamol.

On the last occasion that Jo and the healthcare assistants were on duty together, an agency nurse was also present because of the workload on the ward. However, Jo still did not help unless she felt it was absolutely necessary. At one time during the evening she left the ward for a break stating that she had left the keys on the shelf in the office. These keys included keys to the controlled drug cupboard and the drugs trolley. Although Jo was entitled to a break from the ward, this was the third she had taken that night and she did not tell the staff where she was going.

The agency nurse was angry that Jo had left the ward without informing her of where she was going and how she could be contacted. Jo also did not tell the

## ACTIVITY 3.4 continued

agency nurse where she could find the keys. A patient then complained of pain and the healthcare assistant asked the agency nurse, who was a registered nurse, if she could give the patient some paracetamol. The agency nurse then questioned the healthcare assistants about the procedure they had been following with Jo.

When Jo eventually returned to the ward, the agency nurse challenged her about the drug administration and leaving the keys in the ward office. Jo was offhand with the agency nurse and did not speak to her for the rest of the shift. At the handover to the day staff, Jo gave the report without involving the rest of the night nursing team. She let the healthcare assistants and the agency nurse write up the nursing records, but at no time in the handover did she involve them in the verbal report.

The agency nurse complained to the ward manager about the incidents that had occurred, and also some problems relating to a blood transfusion that Jo had been managing. It appeared that Jo had not followed the trust protocol with regard to administration of a transfusion. There had been a long delay before it had been commenced and Jo had not recorded any observations of the patient during the transfusion.

### *Conclusion*

An investigation was carried out by the Trust and it was felt that Jo should be dismissed from her post and her case referred to the Nursing and Midwifery Council. Jo was charged by the NMC and found guilty of:

- failing to provide adequate support for patients on a ward;
- giving medication to healthcare assistants to administer to patients;
- leaving a ward without advising staff of her whereabouts, and not handing over the ward keys to a registered nurse colleague;
- failing to provide an adequate and appropriate handover of patient care;
- failing to follow the correct protocol and procedure while administering a blood transfusion.

Her name was removed from the nursing register.

Note: this case is part of a series based on true cases which were reported to the NMC. Compiled by George Castledine, Professor and Consultant of General Nursing, University of Central England, Birmingham, and Dudley Group of Hospitals NHS Trust.

- you must make it known and obtain help and supervision from a competent practitioner if you feel an aspect of practice lies beyond your level of competence or outside your area of registration.

As previously identified, *The Code* (NMC, 2008a) is divided into sections. The following pages look at some of the issues *The Code* raises in more detail, those of consent, confidentiality, record keeping and maintaining professional knowledge and competence.

## Consent

Every mentally competent adult has the right in law to consent to any touching of his/her person, or to refuse any examination or treatment. If he/she is touched without consent or other lawful justification, then the person has the right to bring a criminal action for battery, or a civil action for trespass to the person (Dimond, 2011). Furthermore, should harm occur to the patient, it could result in a legal action against the nurse for negligence. Consent also affirms the person's right to self-determination and autonomy (Caulfield, 2005). Lord Donaldson, once the second most senior judge in England and Wales, pointed out that consent is twofold – first to obtain 'legal' justification for care (as above), and secondly 'clinical' consent to secure the patient's trust and co-operation.

The NMC (2008a, clause 13) states that as a registered nurse 'you must ensure that you gain consent before any treatment or care'. It also states that it is a professional duty that any information given to the patient to help them make an informed decision must be accurate and truthful and presented in such a way as to be easily understood.

Consent can be written, verbal or implied ('by co-operation'). They are all equally valid. However, they vary considerably in their value as evidence in proving that consent was given. Consent in writing is the best form of evidence and therefore is the preferred method for patients when any procedure involving some risk is contemplated. As a student you would not be expected to give information to patients about their condition or treatment or to obtain any written consent. However, any form of nursing intervention requires the patient's consent. When referring to students the NMC (2011a, p. 14) points out that you must:

- make sure people know that you are a student;

- ensure that you gain their consent before you begin to provide care;

- respect the right for people to request care to be provided by a registered professional.

It is a basic principle of law in this country that a mentally competent adult has the right to refuse treatment and take his or her own discharge contrary to medical advice. The NMC (2008a, clause 14) supports this by stating that 'you must respect and support people's rights to accept or decline treatment and care'.

Consent must be:

- given by a legally competent person;
- informed;
- given freely.

## A legally competent person

The person giving consent must have the capacity to do so. A legally competent person must be able to understand and retain information and use the information to make an informed decision. You must presume that a patient is competent unless otherwise assessed by a suitably qualified practitioner. The assessment of whether an adult lacks the capacity to consent is made by the clinician providing treatment or care, but it should involve nurses' views as well.

No one has the right to consent on behalf of another competent adult. Further, it is accepted that adults over the age of 16 have the relevant capacity to understand and make their own decisions about medical and nursing treatment (Caulfield, 2005).

### Adults temporarily unable to consent

In emergency situations where an adult becomes unable to consent (for example, if they are unconscious), the law allows treatment as long as it is 'in the patient's best interests'. Medical intervention that can be delayed until the patient can consent should be delayed (exceptions to this are if the person has issued an advanced directive refusing treatment, in which case the treatment is not given). In 'the patient's best interests' is said to be when a 'body of other similar treatment providers would also give the same treatment' (Tingle and Cribb, 2007, p. 168), and arises from a court case in 1989 (*F. v. West Berkshire Health Authority*).

## Informed consent

The patient must be able to give informed consent to the proposed treatments, and the information given by any health care professional (including registered nurses) should include any material risks such as the nature and consequences of the proposed treatment, the consequences of not having the treatment and any alternatives to the treatment.

## Given freely

Consent must be given freely – this means that no threats or implied threats must be used, that no 'coercion and undue influence' is applied. Coercion invalidates consent, and if a nurse feels that the patient is being coerced, either by another health care professional or by a family member, they should seek to see the patient alone to ascertain that *their* wishes are being adhered to (Peate, 2006).

## Children and young people

If the patient is under 18 years old (age of consent) the rules concerning consent for medical treatment are different. A person aged 16–17 is allowed to consent to treatment under the Family Law Reform Act (1979), in a similar way to an adult. However, *refusal* of treatment can be overridden by a person with parental authority or a court order until they are 18 years old.

A person under the age of 16 years, who has sufficient understanding and intelligence to enable them to understand the proposed treatment or investigation *may* have the capacity to consent (Department of Health, 2009). Children who have these capacities are said to be 'Gillick competent'. The term Gillick (sometimes referred to as 'Fraser' after the judge who heard the case) comes from a court case in 1985 which concerned a teenage girl's right to consent to medical treatment without her parents' knowledge (*Gillick* v. *West Norfolk and Wisbech Area Health Authority*).

An assessment to determine whether a minor is Gillick (Fraser) competent must consider the following questions (Peate, 2006, p. 72):

- Does the child understand the proposed treatment, his/her medical condition, and the consequences that may emerge if he/she refuses or agrees to treatment?

- Does he/she understand the moral, social and family issues involved in the decision he/she is to make?

- Does the mental state of the child fluctuate?

- What treatment is to be performed? Does the child understand the complexities of the proposed treatment and the potential risks associated with it?

# Mental Capacity Act (2005)

The Mental Capacity Act affects people living in England and Wales over the age of 16. It is concerned with protecting people who lack the capacity to make their own decisions about a variety of health and social circumstances.

The Act includes:

- a test to determine 'a person's best interests';

- Lasting Powers of Attorney that extend to a person's health and welfare as well as property and money;

- a Court of Protection and an office of Public Guardian to support the Court;

- deputies who can make decisions in the 'person's best interests';

- a criminal offence of ill-treatment and neglect;

- regulation of advance decisions to refuse treatment;

- regulation of research in relation to individuals who lack mental capacity;

- an Independent Mental Capacity Advocate service (IMCA) for people with no family or friends;

- a Code of Practice to accompany the Act – health care professionals have a duty to abide by the Code.

## Underlying principles of the Mental Capacity Act (2005)

- A presumption of capacity: everyone has the right to make their own decisions, so a person must be assumed to have capacity unless it is established that they lack capacity.

- Individuals should be supported where possible so that they can make their own decisions: a person must not be treated as being unable to make a decision unless all practicable steps to help them to do so have been taken, without success.

- People have the right to make decisions which may seem eccentric or unwise to other people: a person is not to be treated as unable to make a clear decision merely because he or she makes an unwise decision.

- Best interests: acts done or decisions made on behalf of a person established to be lacking capacity must be in their best interests.

- Rights and freedoms must be restricted as little as possible: before doing an act or taking a decision on behalf of a person, regard must be had as to whether the purpose underlying that act or decision can be achieved in a way that is less restrictive of his rights or freedom of action.

A person who lacks capacity:

- is unable to make a decision for themselves by reason of disturbance of their mind or brain, whether on a temporary or permanent basis;

- is unable to make a decision if they cannot understand relevant information, retain that information, use or weigh that information as part of making a decision, or is unable to communicate their decision 'by any means'.

Lack of capacity cannot be established merely by reference to a person's age, appearance or behaviour.

(www.justice.gov.uk)

### Advance decisions to refuse treatment

The Mental Capacity Act (2005) allows adults over the age of 18 years to state, in writing, in advance what treatment they would *not* like carried out should they become unable to give consent. These decisions must be respected by all health care professionals, including nurses. The person must be deemed competent when making the advance directive, and only clear refusals of specific treatments will be upheld (surgery, drug therapy, etc). If any doubt exists, then treatment may be given 'in the patient's best interests'. Furthermore, a patient cannot refuse basic care.

### Mental Health Acts

For people detained under relevant mental health legislation, the principles of consent continue to apply for all conditions not related to the mental disorder.

### FURTHER INFORMATION

Further information about consent can be obtained from the Department of Health website at www.dh.gov.uk (type 'consent' in the main search engine).

Key guidance includes:

- reference guide to consent for examination or treatment;

- good practice in consent implementation guide.

In addition, on the same website, there is information about consent forms and associated guidance for patients. Another website with information about the Mental Capacity Act (2005) is the Department of Justice (www.justice.gov.uk).

# Confidentiality

Confidentiality is a fundamental part of the patient/carer relationship. Any information given to a nurse by a patient should not be passed on to anyone outside the health care team without the patient's consent. The fundamental importance of trust between a health professional and the patient brings with it a 'duty of confidence' (Caulfield, 2005).

This duty arises from:

- duty of care in negligence (discussed earlier in the chapter) – a breach of confidentiality can lead to civil action;

- implied duties under the nurse's contract of employment;

- requirements of the NMC outlined in *The Code* – a breach of this could result in removal from the nurses' register.

The NMC endorses Caulfield's statements in *The Code* by stating (NMC, 2008a, clauses 5–6):

- you must respect people's right to confidentiality;

- you must ensure people are informed about how and why information is shared by those who will be providing care.

## Disclosing information

Although *The Code* requires you to respect patient confidentiality, it also states:

- you must disclose information if you believe someone may be at risk of harm, in line with the law of the country in which you are practising.

(NMC, 2008a, clause 7)

However, disclosure of confidential information without consent should only happen in exceptional circumstances. Nurses must be able to justify their actions in doing so, and it must only be done in the public interest to protect individuals, groups or society as a whole from the risk of significant harm. Examples could include child abuse, serious crime or drug trafficking. If a decision to disclose is made, a clear and accurate account should be recorded in the person's records.

Dimond (2011) summarises this when stating there are seven exceptions to the duty of confidence, when nurses can divulge information about their patients:

- with the patient's consent;
- in the patient's best interests;
- by court order;
- under a statutory duty to disclose;
- in the public interests;
- to the police;
- under provisions within the Data Protection Act (1998).

Confidentiality does not only apply within a health care setting. As a student you may wish to refer to a real-life situation you have been involved with in an academic assignment. If so, your university will have guidelines on confidentiality that you must abide by, which will advise you not to provide any information that could identify a particular patient.

## Ownership of and access to records

Records of information belong to an organisation (for example, a hospital) and not to specific people. People can, however, request to see their paper-held and computer-held notes, usually on payment of a fee, under the following Acts:

- The Data Protection Act 1998 gives the patient a statutory right to access personal information in the form of health records held on them (both computer and manually-held records). The definition of 'health record' includes all records relating to their health, such as nursing records, physiotherapy records, laboratory results, etc. The patient also has the right of rectification, that is, correcting or amending the data recorded, if they appear to be inaccurate.

- The Access to Medical Reports Act 1988 gives an individual the right of access to any medical report relating to them which is supplied for employment or insurance purposes.

- The Access to Health Records Act 1990 governs access to health records of deceased people.

- The Freedom of Information Act 2000 and Freedom of Information (Scotland) Act 2002 grant anyone the right to information held by public authorities that is not covered by the Data Protection Act 1998.

## Caldicott Guardians

A review was commissioned in 1997 by the Chief Medical Officer of England in response to:

> increasing concern about the ways in which patient information is being used in the NHS in England and Wales and the need to ensure that confidentiality is not undermined. Such concern was largely due to the development of information technology in the service, and its capacity to disseminate information about patients rapidly and extensively.
>
> (Department of Health, 1999)

As a result of the report every NHS organisation is required to appoint a 'Caldicott Guardian' who is responsible for agreeing and reviewing internal protocols governing the protection and use of patient-identifiable information by the staff of their organisations.

---

**FURTHER INFORMATION**

- Further information about confidentiality can be obtained from the Department of Health website at www.dh.gov.uk (type 'confidentiality NHS code of practice' in the main search engine).

- Key guidance includes:

  - what is confidential information?;

  - providing a confidential service;

  - legal requirements;

  - a list of confidentiality decisions.

# Record keeping

Record keeping is part of the professional duty of care owed by the registered nurse to the patient. As a student you can take part in record keeping activities provided you have the knowledge and skills to undertake this and you are adequately supervised. Your ability to contribute to record keeping will be assessed in your practice area by the person delegating the task to you (usually your mentor) – if they feel you are not competent they must clearly countersign any entries made by you.

The NMC states this in its *Record Keeping: Guidance for Nurses and Midwives* (2009):

> Record keeping is an integral part of nursing, midwifery and specialist community public health nursing practice. It is a tool of professional practice and one that should help the care process. It is not separate from this process and it is not an optional extra to be fitted in if circumstances allow.
>
> (NMC, 2009, p. 1)

The NMC (2009, p. 12) further says that good record keeping helps to protect the welfare of patients / clients by:

- helping to improve accountability;

- showing how decisions related to patient care were made;

- supporting the delivery of services;

- supporting effective clinical judgements and decisions;

- supporting patient care and communications;

- making continuity of care easier;

- providing documentary evidence of services delivered;

- promoting better communication and sharing of information between members of the multi-professional health care team;

- helping to identify risks, and enabling early detection of complications;

- supporting clinical audit, research, allocation of resources and performance planning;

- helping to address complaints or legal processes.

Patients should be equal partners, whenever possible, in the completion of their records. They have the right to expect that all health care professionals, including registered nurses and student nurses who contribute to their records, will practise a high standard of record keeping. Therefore, failure on the part of a registered nurse to maintain reasonable standards of record keeping could be evidence of professional misconduct and subject to Fitness to Practise proceedings. Records can also be called as evidence by the Health Services Commissioner, before a court of law, or in a local investigation of a complaint made by a patient. This may include anything that makes reference to a patient such as:

• handwritten clinical notes;

• emails;

• letters to and from other health professionals;

• laboratory reports;

• X-rays;

• printouts from monitoring equipment;

• incident reports and statements;

• photographs;

• videos;

• recordings of telephone conversations;

• text messages.

Any absence of a record may be seen as a lack of care, negligence, inability to write a record, lack of interest, concealment or a general failure to communicate in the best interest of the patient. A coroner stated: 'Nurses are good observers - it's only a question of whether or not they write their observations down – when they come to court to testify, facts which seemed trivial at the time take on a paramount importance' (anon).

All nurses need to be familiar with the NMC guidelines which can be accessed at www.nmc-uk.org. The salient points of its guidelines are listed below:

## Content and style

The principles of good record keeping include:
1. Handwriting should be legible.
2. All entries to records should be signed. In the case of written records, the person's name and job title should be printed alongside the first entry.
3. In line with local policy, you should put the date and time on all records. This should be in real time and chronological order, and be as close to the actual time as possible.
4. Your records should be accurate and recorded in such a way that the meaning is clear.
5. Records should be factual and not include unnecessary abbreviations, jargon, meaningless phrases or irrelevant speculation.
6. You should use your professional judgement to decide what is relevant and what should be recorded.
7. You should record details of any assessments and reviews undertaken, and provide clear evidence of the arrangements you have made for future and ongoing care. This should also include details of information given about care and treatment.
8. Records should identify any risks or problems that have arisen and show the action taken to deal with them.
9. You have a duty to communicate fully and effectively with your colleagues, ensuring that they have all the information they need about the people in your care.
10. You must not alter or destroy any records without being authorised to do so.
11. In the unlikely event that you need to alter your own or another health care professional's records, you must give your name and job title, and sign and date the original documentation. You should make sure that the alterations you make, and the original record, are clear and auditable.
12. Where appropriate, the person in your care, or their carer, should be involved in the record keeping process.
13. The language that you use should be easily understood by the people in your care.
14. Records should be readable when photocopied or scanned;
15. You should not use coded expressions of sarcasm or humorous abbreviations to describe the people in your care;
16. You should not falsify records.

(NMC, 2009, p. 4)

# Maintaining professional knowledge and competence

Once you are a registered nurse you will have to undertake post-registration education and practice (Prep). This is a set of NMC professional standards and guidance designed to help nurses provide the best possible care for patients and keep up to date with developments in practice by thinking and reflecting on their practice (NMC, 2011b).

In order to renew registration every year registered nurses must provide a signed Notification of Practice (NOP), which asks them, amongst other things, to declare that they have met the Prep requirements. There are two separate Prep standards which affect registration (NMC, 2011b, p. 5):

- **The Prep (practice) standard** – nurses must have worked in some capacity by virtue of their nursing or midwifery qualification for a minimum of 450 hours during the previous three years, or have successfully undertaken an approved return to practice course within the last three years;

- **The Prep (continuing professional development) standard** – nurses must have undertaken and recorded their continuing professional development (CPD) over the three years prior to the renewal of their registration.

Continuing professional development is defined as:

> A process of lifelong learning for all individuals which meets the needs of patients and delivers health outcomes and health care priorities of the NHS which enables professionals to expand and fulfil their potential.
>
> (HSC, 1999/194).

Although this definition specifically refers to the NHS, it applies to all areas where registered nurses are employed.

To satisfy the Prep CPD standard (NMC, 2011b, p. 9) registered nurses must produce evidence that they:

- have undertaken at least 35 hours of learning activity relevant to their practice during the three years prior to renewal of registration;

- have maintained a personal professional profile (PPP) of their learning activity;

- comply with any request from the NMC to audit how these requirements have been met.

For further details on how to meet the Prep requirements see *The Prep Handbook* (2011) at www.nmc-uk.org.

## Providing care in an emergency situation outside the work environment

The NMC (2008b) has issued an advice sheet on providing care in an emergency situation outside the workplace. This spans all the areas of accountability registered nurses are concerned with (criminal, civil, employment and professional law), and as a student you should be aware of the implications for you.

In the United Kingdom there is generally no *legal* obligation on a person to provide care or assistance in an emergency situation. However, in an emergency, in or outside the work setting registered nurses have a *professional* duty to provide care. The NMC points out (NMC, 2008b) that in providing emergency care, registered nurses are personally accountable for any actions or omissions in their practice, and would be judged against what could reasonably be expected from someone with their knowledge, skills and abilities when placed in those circumstances. The registered nurse would need to ensure that this is within the limits of their competence and that they are able to demonstrate that they acted in the person's best interests (NMC, 2008b).

The NMC also acknowledges that student nurses may be placed in emergency situations on occasion; their advice is that 'you recognize and stay within the limits of your competence' and that 'you should work only under the appropriate supervision and support of a qualified professional and ask for help from your mentor or tutor when you need it' in an emergency situation (NMC, 2011a, p. 15).

## And finally.....

Listed below are some of the common reasons why registered nurses are removed from the NMC register. Removal from the register is a result of the findings of Fitness to Practise panels where registered nurses' conduct and performance are measured against *The Code* (NMC, 2008a). Anyone has the right to complain to the NMC about a registered nurse – fellow registered nurses, colleagues in other health care professions, patients and their families, employers, managers and the police. Grounds for removal include:

- failure to provide adequate care;
- failure to protect/promote the interest of patients;
- deliberately concealing unsafe practice;
- failure to act, knowing that a colleague or subordinate is improperly treating or abusing patients;
- committing criminal offences;
- failure to keep proper records, falsifying records;
- continued lack of competence despite opportunities to improve;
- physical or verbal abuse of patients;
- failure to administer medicines safely;
- theft from patients or employers;
- drug-related offences;
- alcohol or drug dependence;
- untreated serious mental illness;
- sexual abuse of patients;
- breach of confidentiality.

Perhaps not on such a serious scale as the above, if you as a student nurse have any doubts about the actions or performance of a registered nurse, you mustn't ignore the situation, even if it could put you in a difficult position. The NMC advises that you challenge the registered nurse as it may help them improve their practice.

**ACTIVITY 3.5**

Visit the NMC website at www.nmc-uk.org/Hearings/Hearings-and-outcomes/ and find details of recent Fitness to Practise cases. Look at the facts of the cases and see how the NMC decided to deal with the allegations.

> **FURTHER READING**
>
> This section has given a very brief introduction to the law. Further detail can be found in a variety of texts written for nurses, perhaps the most comprehensive being Bridgit Dimond's *Legal Aspects of Nursing,* and Helen Caulfield's *Accountability* (see reference list). The following websites are also useful:
>
> British Medical Council www.bma.org.uk
>
> Department of Justice www.justice.gov.uk (Mental Capacity Act)
>
> Department of Health www.dh.gov.uk
>
> European Court of Human Rights www.echr.coe.int
>
> General Medical Council www.gmc-uk.org
>
> Health Service Ombudsman www.ombudsman.org.uk
>
> Information Commission www.ico.gov.uk
>
> Law Society for England and Wales (has a useful section on clinical negligence) www.lawsociety.org.uk
>
> Nursing and Midwifery Council www.nmc-uk.org
>
> Royal College of Nursing www.rcn.org.uk

## Chapter summary

- Registered nurses are accountable in the criminal courts, the civil courts, before their employer and before the Fitness to Practise Committees of the NMC.

- Student nurses are similarly responsible to the criminal courts, civil courts, their university and placement provider and must act within the NMC's *Guidance on Professional Conduct for Nursing and Midwifery Students* (NMC, 2011a).

- Department of Health and NMC guidance for gaining consent, ensuring confidentiality and record keeping must be adhered to.

- Nurses must engage in continuing professional development throughout their working lives.

## References

Banks, S. (2004) *Ethics, Accountability and the Social Professions.* Basingstoke: Palgrave.

Castledine, G. (1991) Accountability in Delivering Care. *Nursing Standard,* **5 (25), 13:** 28–30.

Caulfield, H. (2005) *Vital Notes for Nurses: Accountability.* Oxford: Blackwell Publishing.

Department of Health (1999) *Caldicott Guardians,* NHS Executive, HSC, 1999/012. London: Department of Health.

Department of Health (2009) *Reference Guide to Consent for Examination or Treatment* (2nd edition). London: Department of Health.

Dimond, B. (2011) *Legal Aspects of Nursing* (6th edition). London: Pearson.

Health Act (1999) www.legislation.gov.uk (accessed 12 December 2012)

HSC (1999/194) *Continuing Professional Development (Quality in the New NHS).* London: Department of Health.

Mental Capacity Act (2005) www.legislation.gov.uk (accessed 20 November 2012)

Nursing and Midwifery Council (2008b) Advice sheet: *Providing Care in an Emergency Situation outside The Workplace.* London: NMC.

Nursing and Midwifery Council (2009) *Record Keeping: Guidance for Nurses and Midwives.* London: NMC.

Nursing and Midwifery Council (2011a) *Guidance on Professional Conduct for Nursing and Midwifery Students.* London: NMC.

Nursing and Midwifery Council (2011b) *The Prep Handbook.* London: NMC.

Nursing and Midwifery Order (2001) www.nmc-uk.org/About-us/legislation/the-order/ (accessed 19 November 2012)

Peate, I. (2006) *Becoming a Nurse in the 21st Century.* Chichester: Wiley.

Richards, A. & Edwards, S. (2008) *A Nurse's Survival Guide to the Ward.* London: Churchill Livingstone.

Tingle, J. & Cribb, A. (2007) *Nursing Law and Ethics* (3$^{rd}$ edition). Oxford: Blackwell.

www.justice.gov.uk (accessed 20 November 2012)

# 04
# VALUES AND HEALTH CARE ETHICS

The aim of this chapter is to outline the theories and principles used in the health care ethics and values debate.

**Learning Outcomes**

On completion of this chapter you should be able to:

- explore the concept of values and patients' rights in nursing;
- briefly describe the ethical theories of deontology and utilitarianism;
- briefly describe the four principles of health care ethics: autonomy, beneficence, non-maleficence and justice.

As you work through this chapter, remember that no amount of reading will equip you with a set of absolute rules to solve all the moral problems you encounter. Tschudin (2003) believes ethics can only be described in terms of principles and never in terms of absolutes, while Aristotle is reputed to have said that 'there is a solution to every problem – the only problem is finding it!'

## Values and rights

Values are a fundamental component of the provision, practice and delivery of health and social care...they are particular kinds of beliefs concerned with the worth of an idea or behaviour and are important in guiding actions, judgments, behaviour and attitudes towards others. In addition they are concerned with the norms, rules, habits, expectations and assumptions that are at the heart of society and form the basis of social interactions and relationships.

(Cuthbert and Quallington, 2008, p.1).

The term 'values' is often linked with the term 'ethics', which, in turn, is often used with the term 'morals'. According to Beauchamp and Childress (2008) morality refers to social conventions about right and wrong human conduct, whereas ethics is a general term referring to both morality and ethical theory. All these terms will be discussed in the following pages.

Values are your personal beliefs that influence how you act and how you judge the actions of other people. Development of your personal moral 'knowledge' and values comes from a variety of sources: your upbringing, gender, class, age, religious/spiritual beliefs, peer groups, culture, education, life experiences – the list could be endless, but the important factor is that all perspectives are personal to you and often change as you progress through life.

Every one of us is influenced by our value system. Values have the potential to motivate and guide our choices and decision-making abilities (Peate, 2006), but personal and professional values may not always be the same. Your values may also differ from those of another nurse, even though you are caring for the same patients. This is because they are personal. Cuthbert and Quallington (2008) give the example of two nurses working on a maternity ward who have very different views on abortion, but who are required to deliver the same professional care.

According to Hope (2004) most of us have 'gut reactions' as to what we think is morally right or wrong in certain situations. However, there are some viewpoints that most of us take into account when evaluating others' actions and behaviour, particularly in professional circumstances and regardless of our personal opinions:

- **Legal** – actions are right if they comply with the law, and wrong if they do not.

- **Professional** – actions are right if they are supported by codes of professional conduct, protocols and evidence-based practice, and wrong if they do not.

- **Religious beliefs** – how does God or religious teaching view the action?

- **Social convention** – does the action conform to acceptable norms of behaviour in society?

- **Practical** – an action is right if it is the easiest and most practical way to achieve the desired aim or intention. Conflict will arise if it goes against any of the above or harms the patient.

Fry and Johnstone (2002) point out that nurses should remember that patients also have their own set of personal values, and this could be a source of potential conflict. In this case they advise that nurses must respect the values of others, but ensure that a balance is achieved in relation to the patients' rights and their own professional duties.

## Patients' rights

Patients' rights are sometimes referred to as entitlements or claims and stem from the premise that individuals are unique and valuable and therefore should be afforded certain rights. These are sometimes described as 'positive rights' and 'negative rights'. Positive rights require society, or another individual, to do something positive in order to fulfil or uphold human and legal rights – for example, health care can only be realised if society ensures that health care systems exist and that the individuals in the system fulfil their duty to provide care. A negative right, sometimes referred to as a 'qualified right', relates to the freedom to do something without interference – for example, freedom of expression, or the freedom to practise one's preferred religion or not to practise a religion at all (Cuthbert and Quallington, 2008).

## Human rights

The major piece of international legislation relating to rights is the Human Rights Act (1998) (see also *Chapter 5*). This Act sets out what every person has a right to expect with regard to fundamental human rights and freedoms regardless of gender, disability, ethnic identity, sexuality or class. It makes it unlawful for public authorities (and therefore nurses) to act in a way which is incompatible with the various articles within the act.

Within the fourteen articles of the Human Rights Act, McHale and Gallagher (2003) differentiate between absolute rights, limited rights and qualified rights. Absolute rights cannot be restricted – for example, Article 2, 'The right to life' and Article 3, 'Prohibition of torture'. Limited rights include such articles as Article 5, 'Right to Liberty and Security', which contains a series of legitimate exceptions, such as the lawful detention of persons for the prevention of spreading of infectious diseases, detention of persons of unsound mind, alcoholics or drug addicts or vagrants, and so on. McHale and Gallagher (2003) also refer to a third group, which they call qualified rights, that are found in Articles 8, 9 and 10 – 'Right to respect for private and family life', 'Freedom of thought, conscience and religion' and 'Freedom of expression' respectively – these fall into the same category as Cuthbert and Quallington's 'negative rights'.

The most pertinent of the fourteen articles to nursing are:

- **Article 8: Right to respect for private and family life, home and correspondence.** This confers the right for each person to live their own life as is reasonable within a democratic society and takes account of the freedoms and rights of others. This right can also include the right to have personal information such as official records, including medical information, kept private and confidential. It also places restrictions on the extent to which any public authority can invade an individual's privacy about their body without their permission. In the health care context this has implications in relation to decisions of consent and refusal of treatment, and confidentiality of patient records.

- **Article 9: Freedom of thought, conscience and religion.** This provides an absolute right for a person to hold the thoughts, positions of conscience or religion of their choice. This includes the right for the person to practise or demonstrate their religion in private or public (as long as it does not interfere with the rights and freedoms of others). In a health care setting this article is particularly applicable in relation to the right of health care professionals to opt out of certain procedures on the basis of conscientious objection; for example, assisting with pregnancy terminations. Equally it applies to patients who refuse treatment on religious grounds, such as Jehovah's Witnesses who may refuse transfusion of blood.

- **Article 14: Freedom from discrimination.** In the context of the Act discrimination is defined as 'treating people in similar situations differently, or those in different situations in the same way, without proper justification' (Department for Constitutional Affairs, 2006, p. 25). Everyone is entitled to equal access to all the rights set out in the Act, regardless of personal status. Discrimination is prohibited on grounds of sex, sexual orientation, age, race, colour, language, religion, disability, political or other opinion, national or social origin, association with a national minority, property, birth (for example, whether a person is born inside or outside of marriage) and marital status.

www.legislation.gov.uk

## Legal rights

These are rights which have to be afforded to patients according to the laws of the land (see also *Chapter 3*). Breaches of these rights include criminal acts such as murder, manslaughter, rape, theft, etc. (all of which nurses have been found guilty of). The infringement of legal rights can also lead to civil cases, for example where an action for negligence results from a breach of duty of care.

## Professional considerations

These are clauses within codes of practice and standards which professionals such as nurses have to adhere to in order to maintain their registration. One of the primary functions of the NMC is to protect the public, and it publishes the standards of professional conduct that the public can expect of a registered practitioner (www.nmc-uk.org). Any member of the public can access the NMC website and read the various standards and guidelines that indicate how they should be treated. In addition to the NMC Code (2008), there are various standards published by both the NMC and the Department of Health concerning issues such as confidentiality, consent, delivering competent care, advocacy and anti-discriminatory practice. They all outline patients' rights in these areas and emphasise the need for nurses to respect the standards. Other publications have statements about privacy, dignity and respect implicit within them – for example, National Service Frameworks, NICE (National Institute of Health and Clinical Excellence) guidelines, the Mental Capacity Act (2005), and so on.

In 2009 the Department of Health issued the NHS Constitution which establishes the principles and values of the NHS in England. It sets out:

> the rights to which patients, public and staff are entitled and pledges which the NHS is committed to achieve, together with responsibilities which the public, patients and staff owe to one another to ensure that the NHS operates fairly and effectively. All NHS bodies and private and third sector providers supplying NHS services will be required by law to take account of this Constitution in their decisions and actions.
>
> (Department of Health, 2009, p.2)

## Respect, dignity and privacy

The concepts of respect, dignity and privacy can be found in many health care professionals' codes of practice. Indeed, the first clause of the NMC *Code* states: 'Make the care of patients your first concern, treating them as individuals and respecting their dignity' (NMC, 2008, p. 1). The words 'dignity' and 'respect' are often used together, in that dignity means being worthy of respect, and that giving a person respect will maintain their dignity. Cuthbert and Quallington (2008) believe nurses should respect everyone as a valued unique individual, and they cite Dillon (1992) as saying respect in care involves:

- a belief in the value of persons as individuals and as members of society;

- treating people in the manner in which you expect to be treated;

- showing consideration for another person's feelings and interests;

- an attitude demonstrating that you value another person.

Respect is shown in many ways – demonstrating a genuine interest in your patients, listening to them, preserving their modesty, addressing the patient by the name they prefer, etc. However, there are other forms of respect that nurses have to acknowledge – 'respect for boundaries' such as the laws associated with consent, confidentiality and within codes of conduct, and 'respect for authority' that you should show to personnel more senior to you.

Physical privacy can be hard to promote in a health care situation, and yet patients may be at their most vulnerable away from their familiar surroundings and yearn for privacy. Many environments do not lend themselves to privacy – for example, mixed sex wards, bedpans behind curtains, personal hygiene needs, etc. However, treating the patient with dignity and respect at these times can go a long way to enhancing care where privacy may be compromised. Remember that privacy also extends to the patient's space and belongings. In their own environment this is relatively easy for people to control, but in a health care setting patients are often unable to limit the power of others to intrude.

Respect and dignity are part of the benchmarks published by the Department of Health (2010) in their document *Essence of Care*. This is a set of guidelines aimed at promoting good person-centred care organised around 'factors' and 'benchmarks', as shown in *Table 4.1*.

### Care Quality Commission

To ensure that these guidelines, and indeed all Department of Health guidelines and standards, are upheld, the government established the Care Quality Commission in 2009. This body is the independent regulator of health and social care in England, and its aim is to make sure better care is provided for everyone, whether in hospital, care homes, people's own homes, or elsewhere. To that end they regulate health and adult social care services

**Table 4.1** *Benchmarks of* Essence of Care (Department of Health, 2010, p. 262)

| Factor | Benchmark |
| --- | --- |
| 1. Attitudes and behaviours | Patients feel that they matter all of the time |
| 2. Personal world and personal identity | Patients experience care in an environment that actively encompasses individual values, beliefs and personal relationships |
| 3. Personal boundaries and space | Patients' personal space is actively promoted by all staff |
| 4. Communicating with staff and patients | Communication between staff and patients takes place in a manner which respects their individuality |
| 5. Privacy of patient and confidentiality of patient information | Patient information is shared to enable care, with their consent |
| 6. Privacy, dignity and modesty | Patients' care actively promotes their privacy and dignity, and protects their modesty |
| 7. Availability of an area for complete privacy | Patients and/or carers can access an area that safely provides privacy |

*Privacy* = Freedom from intrusion

*Dignity* = Being worthy of respect

provided by the NHS, local authorities, private companies and voluntary organisations (see also *Chapter 6*).

---

**ACTIVITY 4.1**

How would you ensure that: 'Patients experience care in an environment that actively encompasses individual values, beliefs and personal relationships' (benchmark 2)? Make brief notes.

---

# Health care ethics

The text in this section was adapted from the work of Ian Donaldson of the School of Health and Social Care, Bournemouth University.

It is important to recognise that every individual will have differing opinions and views, and sometimes there are no right or wrong attitudes or beliefs. Burnard and Chapman (2003) note that the term 'ethics' is notoriously ambiguous, conjuring up different images for different people. However, everyone should be able to express their views, while remembering not to exclude alternative viewpoints. Ethical debate is about individuals reflecting on their own and others' viewpoints with insight and reasoning.

Nurses are often confronted with moral dilemmas – this is when they recognise that they both ought and ought not to perform a particular action as there are equally compelling reasons for and against it. This is made increasingly difficult when nurses have differing views and values, often causing disagreements between colleagues or with patients. Griffith and Tengnah (2008) give the example of a nurse who believes a doctor's decision not to resuscitate a patient with a terminal illness is wrong – the nurse believes the patient's life should be sustained, and is suddenly faced with a dilemma about what is right or wrong. Both decisions are lawful, so the decision is one of morality. Another good example of this can be found in the constant debate about abortion – whose rights prevail?

Using theories and principles may help to guide moral deliberations. There are a wide range of differing moral standpoints but three particular ways of moral reasoning have been extremely influential in the shaping and discussions of health care ethics. They are the theories of utilitarianism, deontology, and the principles of health care ethics.

## Utilitarianism

This idea was first put forward by Jeremy Bentham in the eighteenth century and refined by John Stuart Mill in the nineteenth century. Mill believed that the way to evaluate what was morally right or wrong was to examine the outcome or 'consequences' of that action – whether the action produces good consequences, and not just whether it was done with good intentions. Mill's golden rule was that actions are right if they promote happiness and wrong if they produce the reverse of happiness. This rule is often abbreviated to 'the greatest happiness or the greatest good to the greatest number' and that 'the end (the consequences) justifies the means (the action taken)'.

An argument against utilitarianism is that it can promote activities that are a selfish pursuit of pleasure at the expense of everyone else. Mill attempted to solve this critique with two additional 'rules'. He said that actions were good if they created the greatest amount of happiness. This argument means that selfish activities that create happiness for one person but unhappiness in a great deal of other people are not acceptable (for example consider how this 'rule' prevents a paedophile from justifying his actions). Mill's second 'rule' was that there is a difference between the quantity and quality of pleasures that cause happiness. He believes that it is better to pursue high quality pleasures, which he describes as intellectual, aesthetic and imaginative, rather than lower quality pleasures which he describes as 'mere animal instincts'.

A major criticism of utilitarianism is that one cannot predict consequences with certainty; utilitarianism is therefore not useful in guiding individuals as to what they ought to do.

Included in the definition of utilitarianism is the 'rightness or wrongness of an action' and whether it furthers the goal of the greatest happiness for the greatest number (Thompson *et al.*, 2006). This can have implications, for example in a common situation nurses face, which is telling the truth. As a nurse you would have to weigh up the consequences as to whether telling the truth would lead to more 'happiness' than 'unhappiness'. In this instance, it can be very difficult to evaluate the potential long-term benefit to the patient (of knowing the truth) versus the short-term distress (of learning bad news). It is for this reason that some prefer not to use a utilitarian approach, preferring instead to explore what is the right thing to do using a different theory. The theory of deontology is examined below.

## Deontology

The theory of deontology was put forward by Kant in the eighteenth century. He believed it is the *action* that is important and not the consequences. Kant was also concerned with the motive and intentions of the individual performing the action, and argued that the action is only morally right if the individual is motivated by goodwill. Kant's theory is often called the dutiful view of morality, where we are bound by duty to act in a particular way, and not to produce certain consequences.

You may consider that certain actions such as being honest, telling the truth and keeping a promise are right and good actions, but how can an individual decide where their duty lies? Kant argues that we know where our duty lies by considering this question: 'Do I want everyone to behave as I am proposing to do in these circumstances?' This he called the 'categorical imperative', or a universal law. An example of this could be to 'always keep a promise' because you would want others to keep their promises to you – this is therefore something that you would want to be a universal law.

Kant's theory of deontology is criticised for the problems it can create when a categorical imperative, such as always telling the truth, is followed in every situation. However, this criticism seems to miss the point on two counts – first, for many the idea that certain actions are right in themselves and ought to be followed is an important part of their view of morality; secondly, it ignores the process by which the truth is told.

It is important to stress that while both these theories of utilitarianism (concerned with the outcome) and deontology (concerned with the motive) are different, they do not always lead to different evaluations of a particular action (Peate, 2006).

## Principles of health care ethics

Beauchamp and Childress wrote their very influential book in the late 1970s (various editions have been produced since), and many nurses refer to this text. They suggest that there are four key principles in healthcare ethics and argue that by examining a dilemma using these principles the nurse will be helped to decide what the right course of action is.

The key principles are:

- respect for Autonomy;
- Beneficence;
- Non-Maleficence;
- Justice.

### Autonomy

Autonomy, also referred to as self-determination or self-rule or simply 'being one's own person', is defined as 'the capacity to think, decide and act on the basis of such thought and decision ... freely and independently without let or hindrance' (Gillon, 1985, p. 6). Autonomy is seen as being increasingly important within health care, and is closely allied to respect for people's choices.

Cuthbert and Quallington (2008, p. 59) suggest that definitions of autonomy often include references to such terms as:

- self-governance;
- independence;

- individuality;

- self-choice / individual choice;

- freedom / freedom of will;

- being one's own person.

Autonomy is linked with many issues in nursing including values, respect and privacy. In terms of values, Beauchamp and Childress (2008) suggest respect for autonomy is based on the general recognition that an individual has unconditional worth with the capacity to determine their own destiny. Dworkin (1988) believes that people know what is best for them, so giving them the right to express their autonomy will contribute to their happiness and wellbeing.

Patients' autonomy can be compromised when they enter a health care setting. What were previously everyday decisions can be taken away from them – what to wear, when to shower, when and what to eat, where and when to sleep. Peate (2006) points out that talking with the patient and their family can ensure that the patient retains as much autonomous decision-making as possible, and this is a key aspect of the nurse's role. Thompson *et al.* (2006) further suggest nurses should actually protect patients who suffer loss of autonomy through illness, injury or mental disorder. Ramsey (1970) states that autonomy entails working to maintain the optimum degree of independence for the patient and sharing knowledge, care and skills in such a way as to empower the patient, thereby avoiding creating and perpetuating dependency. This, in essence, is allowing the patient freedom to make their own decisions and express their personal preferences and aspirations.

The NMC *Code* (2008) upholds the patient's right to autonomy in many ways – it advocates confidentiality, consent, privacy and dignity among other important issues concerned with autonomy. Dworkin (1988) considers these (particularly consent) and states that the patient's autonomy depends on certain conditions:

- the ability to make independent choices;

- adequate information;

- adequate knowledge.

For example, it is well recognised in this country that any mentally competent adult has the right in law to consent to any touching of his or her person (the law relating to children giving consent is different). For an individual to give consent, and so exercise their autonomy, it is clear that information is required to enable an informed decision to be made. Equally adults have the right to refuse treatment.

### ACTIVITY 4.2

How free are you to make choices? To what extent are you an autonomous person? Think of the last time you made a choice – did you really have total autonomy or were there things that stood in the way? (from Peate, 2006, p. 54)

Paternalism

When an individual acts to override someone's autonomy by restricting information or choices, it is described as paternalism. This is done with the intention of benefiting that person but it takes away their choice (for example, a doctor advocating surgery when the patient does not want an operation). It is always very difficult to know the right course of action in this type of situation. A guide could be to remember that respect for autonomy is of central importance when considering a patient's request, and to ask yourself two questions. First, is the patient mentally competent or is there a situation where a patient's capacity to make an informed decision will compromise their autonomy? Secondly, does the consideration rest on whether one of the other principles (beneficence, non-maleficence or justice) carries greater weight in the particular situation? It is also useful to refer to the NMC *Code* (2008) which is very clear about the nurse's role in gaining consent.

### *Beneficence*

Beneficence is the duty to do good and avoid doing harm to others (both physically and psychologically), and has been described as 'do unto others as you would have them do unto you' (Thompson *et al.*, 2006). As a nurse you have a duty of care to your patients (NMC, 2008) and a duty to promote what is best for your patients. This has been the guiding principle in health care for some time, and is accomplished by acting in the patient's 'best interests'.

However, acting in the patient's best interests raises the question of who should be the judge of what is best for the patient (Hope, 2004). Linked with the principle of autonomy, it should be the patient who decides, but in some instances this is not possible. The Mental Capacity Act (2005) recognises this and is concerned with protecting those who lack the capacity to make their own decisions or consent to treatment in a variety of health and social circumstances – this can either be on a temporary or permanent basis (see *Chapter 3*). The NMC (2008, clause 17) highlights this in the *Code* when talking about temporary inability to make decisions: 'You must be able to demonstrate that you have acted in someone's best interests if you have provided care in an emergency'.

The principle of beneficence can cause tensions if a competent patient decides on an action which is not in their best interests (for example, a Jehovah's Witness refusing a life-saving blood transfusion), where, if action was taken, the hospital staff would be 'violating the bodily integrity of the person without consent' (Hope, 2004), which in legal terms would amount to committing battery.

Seedhouse (2009) includes truth-telling in his discussion of beneficence, and believes it is a central principle of conduct. However, he also believes there are some instances when it is better not to tell the truth, thereby propounding the principle of non-maleficence. He gives the example of allowing patients to read their medical records. Truth-telling relates closely to respect for the person and their autonomy, particularly when it comes to giving information on which people will base their choices and decisions in health and care (Cuthbert and Quallington, 2008). Indeed the NMC (2008) state that patients are entitled to accurate and *truthful* information which is presented in a way they can understand.

---

**ACTIVITY 4.3**

Consider a situation from your placements when information was withheld.

- Was this justified?
- What ethical, legal and professional implications arose from this type of action?
- How was the situation resolved?
- Do you think this was satisfactory – if not, why not?

---

## Non-maleficence

This principle states 'above all to do no harm', which has been likened to the opposite of beneficence, but it is not quite the same thing as many nursing interventions may cause harm. However, it is clear that to intentionally cause distress is morally wrong. Beauchamp and Childress (2008) point out that obligations not to harm are sometimes more stringent than obligations to help, and the NMC endorses this in *The Code* (2008) when it states that in caring for patients, nurses must provide a safe standard of care that avoids or minimises risks (NMC, 2008). Apart from the ethical aspects of this, failure to comply could bring a court action for negligence.

### ACTIVITY 4.4

Can you think of a situation where harm could be caused to a patient, but in the long term it would be in their best interests?

### *Justice*

The final principle to consider is that of justice – that 'everyone is valued equally and treated alike' (Peate, 2006, p. 57). According to Hope (2004, p. 66) there are four elements to this principle:

• **Distributive justice** (sometimes termed entitlement): patients in similar situations should normally have access to the same health care and, in determining what level of health care should be available for one set of patients, account should be taken of the effect of such a use of resources on other patients. In other words, limited resources should be distributed fairly.

• **Respect for the law**: the fact that an act is, or is not, within the law is of moral relevance. Some people may take the view that it might be, in some situations, morally right to break the law, but laws are made through a democratic process and have to be enforced.

• **Rights**: the fundamental idea that a person has rights is a safeguard to their rights being respected, even if overall the social good is thereby diminished.

• **Retributive justice**: concerns the fitting of punishment to the crime – an element not really concerned with health care provision.

When considering distributive justice or 'entitlement', there is a range of different options for the allocation of resources in health care:

• equal share to everyone;

• random distribution;

- on a first come, first served basis;

- according to need;

- to deserving cases;

- to treat as many as possible.

Some of these options can in themselves create inequalities. For example, to allocate an equal share of a resource to everyone may in some cases be perceived as wrong because some individuals are disadvantaged as they have a greater need.

> **FURTHER READING**
>
> *Values for Care Practice* by Sue Cuthbert and Jan Quallington provides a detailed exploration of health care values.

## Chapter summary

- The words values, ethics and morals are often used interchangeably.

- Different viewpoints shape individuals' behaviour towards each other.

- Everyone has fundamental rights under the Human Rights Act.

- Respect, dignity and privacy are key concepts when delivering nursing care.

- Principles of health care ethics should be considered when caring for patients.

## References

Beauchamp, T. and Childress, J. (2008) *Principles of Biomedical Ethics* (6th edition). Oxford: Oxford University Press.

Burnard, P. & Chapman, C. (2003) *Professional and Ethical Issues in Nursing* (3rd edition). London: Bailliere Tindall.

Cuthbert, S. & Quallington, J. (2008) *Values and Care Practice*. Exeter: Reflect Press.

Department for Constitutional Affairs (2006) *A Guide to the Human Rights Act 1998* (3rd edition). London: DCA.

Department of Health (2009) *The NHS Constitution*. London: Department of Health.

Department of Health (2010) *Essence of Care: Patient-focused Benchmarking for Health Care Practitioners*. London: HMSO.

Department of Health (2005) *The Mental Capacity Act*. London: HMSO.

Dillon, R. (1992) Respect and care: toward moral integration. *Canadian Journal of Philosophy*, **(22):** 105–32, in: Cuthbert, S. & Quallington, J. (2008) *Values and Care Practice*. Exeter: Reflect Press.

Dworkin, G. (1988) *The Theory and Practice of Autonomy*. New York: Cambridge University Press.

Fry, S. & Johnstone, M. (2002) *Ethics in Nursing Practice: A Guide to Ethical Decision Making*. Oxford: Blackwell, in: Peate, I. (2006) *Becoming a Nurse in the 21ˢᵗ Century*, Chichester: Wiley.

Gillon, R. (1985) *Philosophical Medical Ethics*. Chichester: Wiley.

Griffith, R. and Tengnah, C. (2008) *Law and Professional Issues in Nursing*. Exeter: Learning Matters.

Hope, T. (2004) *Medical Ethics: A Very Short Introduction*. Oxford: Oxford University Press.

McHale, J. and Gallagher, A. (2003) *Nursing and Human Rights*. Edinburgh: Butterworth Heinemann.

Nursing and Midwifery Council (2008) *The Code: Standards of Conduct, Performance and Ethics for Nurses and Midwives*. London: NMC.

Peate, I. (2006) *Becoming a Nurse in the 21ˢᵗ Century*, Chichester: Wiley.

Ramsey, P. (1970) *The Patient as Person*. New Haven: Yale University Press.

Seedhouse, D. (2009) *The Heart of Healthcare*. Chichester: Wiley.

Thompson, I., Melia, K., Boyd, K., & Horsburgh, D. (2006) *Nursing Ethics* (5th edition). Edinburgh: Churchill Livingstone.

Tschudin, V. (2003) *Ethics in Nursing: The Caring Relationship*. London: Butterworth Heinemann.

www.nmc-uk.org (accessed 20 November 2012)

www.legislation.gov.uk (accessed 20 November 2012)

# 05
# THE UK AS A CULTURALLY DIVERSE SOCIETY

The aim of this chapter is to explore briefly the concept of culture and to raise your awareness of cultural considerations relating to the delivery of health care within a culturally diverse society.

| **Learning Outcomes** | • discuss the concept of culture and understand the associated terminology; |
|---|---|
| On completion of this chapter you should be able to: | • appraise the customs and factors that may have an impact on the provision, delivery and receipt of health care for some service users; |
| | • reflect on your own personal experiences of the multicultural dimensions of care; |
| | • outline key issues associated with transcultural care; |
| | • outline current legislation important to practice. |

## Introduction

The population of Britain, like that of many European countries, has been shaped considerably by post-war patterns of emigration and immigration. According to the Office for National Statistics, the 2011 Census highlights the fact that there continues to be an increasing number of people identifying with minority ethnic groups in the United Kingdom (UK). Within England and Wales a total of seventeen differing ethnic groups were recorded (including 'Other White'), representing approximately 19% of the overall population in these two regions. Given this information it is easy to understand why the UK is now considered to be a multicultural, multiethnic and multifaith society (www.ons.gov.uk).

## Culture

According to Macionis and Plummer (2008, p. 128), culture encompasses 'the values, beliefs, behaviour, practices and material objects that constitute a people's way of life'. It includes such factors as how they dress, their marriage customs and family life, their patterns of work, religious ceremonies and leisure pursuits. It is also perceived as a bridge to the past as well as a guide to the future. A review of the literature, for example, Papadopoulous (2006), Andrews and Boyle (2007), and Jirwe (2008), identifies four main characteristics of culture:

1. **It is learned** from birth through the process of language acquisition and socialisation. From society's point of view, socialisation is the way culture is transmitted and the individual is fitted into the group's organised way of life.
2. **It is shared** by all members of the same cultural group; in fact it is the sharing of cultural beliefs and patterns that binds people together under one identity as a group (even though this is not always a conscious process).
3. **It is an adaptation** to specific activities related to environmental and technical factors and to the availability of natural resources.
4. **It is a dynamic, ever changing process**. People do not merely receive their culture from others, they also make it and remake it continually in a process of interaction with others.

Hofstede and Hofstede (2004) also identify numerous layers of culture which include:

- national;
- regional;
- gender;
- generational;
- professional;
- organisational;
- social class.

Finally, Geiger and Davidhizar (2007) suggest the following cultural phenomena exist:

- **Communication** – there is no known culture without a grammatically complex language, with different languages having different meanings.

- **Social organisation** – family systems and religious and other organisation groups vary among cultures.

- **Space** – various cultures have different concepts about social, personal space and territory.

- **Time** – each culture has its own conception and orientation of time.

- **Environmental control** – the values, beliefs and concepts of health practices vary widely among cultural groups. If it is not easy to understand the logic of a particular belief or practice, that does not mean there is no logic behind it; it need not be logically based on the laws of Western medical science to be valid and practical.

- **Biological considerations** – constitutional endowment and vulnerability differ among people representing different cultures.

## Associated cultural terminology

Terminology closely associated with the term 'culture' includes the terms ethnicity, ethnocentrism and race.

### Ethnicity

There does not appear to be a single, universally accepted concept of ethnicity and this in itself can pose problems for nurses caring for patients from diverse multi-ethnic groups. It is generally perceived as a term that represents a given social group with a shared history, sense of identity, country of origin, language, religion and cultural practices that characterise and distinguish them from other groups. Ethnic differences are wholly learnt and a result of socialisation and acculturation.

### Ethnocentrism

According to Macionis and Plummer (2008, p. 140) this term refers to 'the practice of judging another culture by the standards of one's own culture' and it can imply the assumption that one's own cultural group is superior to that of others. Clearly, to adopt such an approach would be totally against providing holistic care to individual patients.

### Race

Klein (1971) suggests the word 'race' may have initially meant 'to unite' or 'to join'. Later it was used more loosely for national groups such as, for example, the French or German race. In the nineteenth century, scientists took it over to describe the 'races of man': groups defined by their physical appearance from one another, in aspects such as skin colour, hair type and body shape, etc. Numerous theories were developed about these different races, which have now long since been discredited as unscientific and wrong. Race is now widely acknowledged as a social/political construct rather than a biological or genetic fact.

However culture and its associated terms are defined, it is important to remember that it includes historical, present and future dimensions and has immense implications for the care you need to provide. Culture is not homogenous and therefore generalisations about individual members from a group should not be made as they can lead to stereotypical attitudes, cultural misunderstanding, prejudices and discrimination (Jirwe, 2008).

## Culture in practice

Given the population profile of the UK, you will inevitably find yourself in the position of caring for patients from a variety of cultural and ethnic backgrounds, which will require you to have an understanding of the knowledge and skills required for effective transcultural nursing.

**ACTIVITY 5.1**

What do you think is meant by the term 'transcultural nursing'?

Leininger and McFarland (2002) suggest that transcultural nursing is theory and practice that focuses specifically on comparing the care for people with differences and similarities in beliefs, values and cultures in order to provide meaningful and beneficial health care. Wagner (2002) suggests that to achieve this requires both health care practitioners and the institution to consider how their practice can guarantee 'recognition, respect and nurturing' of the individual patient's cultural identity. Gerrish *et al.* (1996, cited in RCN, 2006) suggest this can involve the need to:

- reflect honestly on your own ethnicity;

- interrogate (both intellectually and emotionally) your response to the reality of ethnicity among your patient group;

- make explicit any implicit attitudes which might impact negatively on the care given to people of different ethnic backgrounds.

They also suggest that nursing professionals need to acquire and develop transcultural 'communicative competence'. Again, at the heart of this lies the capacity for 'adaptability in the sense that the practitioner is able to suspend or modify their own cultural expectations and accommodate new cultural demands…'. This requires the nurse to learn and understand the cultural values, behavioural patterns and interaction in specific cultures.

It is also worth remembering that the Nursing and Midwifery Council Code (2008) identifies that you must:

> Make the care of people your first concern, treating them as individuals and respecting their dignity – you must not discriminate in any way against those in your care… (section 1:2)

> Be open and honest, act with integrity and uphold the reputation of your profession – you must demonstrate a personal and professional commitment to equality and diversity (section 4:48)

This means that every practitioner should seek to ensure that they provide and deliver care that meets the religious, dietary and linguistic requirements of patients, whilst ensuring that the principle of individualised care is not compromised.

The following brief notes seek to remind you or raise your awareness of some differing cultural /spiritual beliefs you may encounter while working as a nurse.

## Christianity

Christians believe in the Holy Trinity of one God, the father of mankind who created heaven and earth, and who sent his son Jesus Christ to save mankind, and then sent the Holy Spirit to continue his work in human affairs. Christians believe that everything is created and given life by God the Father. Christianity stresses the importance of living a good life in response to God's love. It encompasses many groups and sects, but the main ones in the UK are the Anglican Church (which includes the Church of England, Church of Wales, Church of Scotland and Church of Ireland), the Roman Catholic Church, the free or non-conformist churches (for example, the Baptist Church, Methodist Church) and the Eastern Orthodox Churches (for example the Greek and Russian Orthodox Churches).

The Christian holy book is the Bible, the interpretation of which can differ between different sects or groups and so has implications for delivery and acceptance of treatment and care. It is therefore very important that you establish from the outset to which Christian sect or group an individual belongs.

### Considerations for practice

Diet

Most Christians do not follow religious dietary restrictions, although some Roman Catholics may wish not to eat meat on Fridays, Ash Wednesday or Good Friday. They should therefore be offered a fish or vegetarian alternative.

Prayers

Some Christians may wish to receive Holy Communion and, possibly, the Anointing of the Sick, which involves being anointed with holy oil. A private and, where possible, quiet area of the care environment should be found if these rituals take place.

Dying and death

Roman Catholics may wish a priest to carry out the sacrament of the 'Last Rites or Extreme Unction' (anointing). If they are able, the individual may also wish to receive Holy Communion and confess their sins to the priest either before receiving Holy Communion or separately. There are no particular rituals associated with last offices.

## Jehovah's Witnesses

Jehovah's Witnesses consider their religion to be a restoration of original first-century Christianity. They accept both the Old and the New Testament of the Bible as inspired by God. They believe in one God 'Jehovah', with the commands in the Bible being very important, and they therefore try to live by them at all times.

### *Considerations for practice*

Jehovah's Witnesses are totally opposed to taking blood or blood products into the body. This means that they will not accept blood transfusions even in life-threatening situations. However, they may accept alternative treatments.

### Diet

Anything that contains blood or blood products is unacceptable, as is meat that has come from an animal that has been strangled, shot or not bled properly. If in doubt, Jehovah's Witnesses should be offered a vegetarian diet.

### Patient confidentiality

Confidentiality must be maintained at all times and the patient's permission must be sought regarding what information they would like to be passed on to their family.

### Death and dying

There are no particular rites and rituals associated with death and dying.

## Hinduism

Originating in northern India, Hinduism is an amalgamation of many local faiths and is inextricably linked to culture and social structure. Hindus believe there is one God who can be worshipped and understood in many different forms. There is a belief in reincarnation in which the status and caste (hereditary or marital social class system) of each life is determined by the behaviour in the last life.

Hinduism does not have one leader, a unified code of conduct or creed. Because of this diversity it is difficult to generalise about what a specific individual might believe.

### *Considerations for practice*

### Physical examination

Generally, Hindu patients will have a strong preference for being treated and cared for by health care staff of the same gender. Privacy during any procedure is very important and female patients may be reluctant to remove clothing. They may also wish for a family member to act as a chaperone when physical examination and procedures are being carried out. Care must be taken not to remove any jewellery, threads, etc. without the patient's / family's permission as they often have a religious significance.

### Personal hygiene

Hindus prefer to shower rather than bathe and should always be provided with water for washing when they go to the toilet.

### Diet

Most Hindus are vegetarian, refusing to take the lives of animals for food. Devout Hindus would not eat off a plate on which meat has been served so an acceptable alternative (for example a plastic or paper plate) might need to be found.

### Medication

Medication that contains animal products should be avoided.

### Family and individual

As Hindus are intimately integrated with their extended family, there may be issues related to decision-making. Often decisions may be taken by a senior member of the family, or a female patient may wish her husband to consent to any treatment on her behalf.

Hindu patients tend to be visited frequently by their extended family, which can cause some difficulties with regard to preset visiting times and the policies concerning numbers of visitors which exist in most hospitals. The family may also wish to perform religious ceremonies with the patient. Privacy should be afforded to allow this to happen.

### Prayer and ritual observance

Devout Hindus pray three times a day (at sunrise, noon and sunset). They should be assisted to wash before prayers if they are unable to do so independently. Where possible a quiet area should be provided and they should not be disturbed during prayer. Patients may wish to have statues or pictures of Gods at their bedside and these items need to be treated with great care and respect.

Dying and death

Death in hospital can cause considerable religious distress to a Hindu patient and their family. Therefore, many patients may have a strong desire, and should be allowed, to die at home. If in hospital they will need to be surrounded by their family who may wish to read passages from holy texts, say prayers with and for them, and perform required ceremonies.

After death real distress may be caused if a non-Hindu touches the body without wearing disposable gloves. Unless otherwise advised by the family, close the eyes and straighten the legs. Do not cut the hair, nails or beard. Hands should be placed on the chest with the palms together and fingers under the chin. Religious objects or jewellery should not be removed. Wrap the body in a plain white sheet.

## Judaism

Jews consider themselves a nation as much as a religious community. The religious aspects of Judaism are based on the relationship between God and man, and relationships between individual humans based on principles of fairness and equality. Religious observance is a means of publicly displaying a personal acceptance of a close connection between the individual and God. Orthodox Jews are very devout in their faith and adhere strictly to the ancient Torah (holy scriptures/laws). Reform or Liberal Jews believe in the Torah but interpret the laws and scriptures in relation to modern-day circumstances.

### *Considerations for practice*

Personal hygiene

Orthodox Jews may wish to wash themselves before and after eating. Running water is required for this, so if the patient is unable to get out of bed, a bowl and jug of water should be offered.

Diet

Only Kosher food is acceptable to many Jewish patients. Milk and meat are not eaten at the same meal. Meat must be killed according to Kosher ritual and is acceptable only from animals which chew the cud and have cloven hooves, or poultry. Pig and rabbit are forbidden. Fish must have fins and scales and therefore shellfish are forbidden. If Kosher meals are not available, a vegetarian diet should be offered.

### Prayer

Jews usually say prayers three times a day and privacy and peace should be given to allow this to happen. The Sabbath is a holy day in which Jews are restricted in what they may do. It begins at sunset on Friday and ends at sunset on Saturday. It is important to establish the patient's principles with regard to the Sabbath as they may significantly impact on the care offered during this time (for example, a patient may not be willing to use a pen to sign their name on forms).

### Death and dying

A Jew who is dying may wish to hear or recite special psalms (particularly Psalm 23).

After death the body should be touched by care staff as little as possible and disposable gloves should be worn at all times. Contact should be made with either the next of kin or the rabbi as soon as possible as they will arrange for the preparation of the body. The face should be covered with a clean cloth or sheet, arms should not be crossed but left at the side of the body with palms facing inwards. Any catheters, drains and tubes should be left in place, as should any wound dressings. Open wounds should be covered. If the patient dies at night the light should be left on when there is no one in the room or bed space. Female bodies should be attended to by female care staff and if at all possible male bodies by male care staff.

## Islam

Islam means 'submission and peace' and includes acceptance of those articles of faith, commands and ordinances revealed through the prophet Mohammed. Muslims follow the Islamic faith and believe that the whole universe is under the direction of Allah and nothing can happen unless he wills it. Most practising Muslims follow five main duties or pillars of Islam:

- faith in one God;

- prayer at five set times every day;

- give a required amount to charity each year;

- fast during the holy month of Ramadan;

- make a pilgrimage (hajj) once in their lives to Mecca if they can.

### Considerations for practice

Physical examination / procedures

Physical examination and procedures should generally be carried out by a member of the health care team of the same gender as the patient. Privacy during any procedure is very important and female patients may be reluctant to remove clothing. They may also wish for a family member to act as a chaperone when physical examination / procedures are being carried out. Consideration should be given to ensure that the patient remains covered appropriately throughout the examination and any other procedure that may need to be performed as part of the care provided. Care must be taken not to remove any jewellery without the patient's / family's permission as it often has a special or religious significance to the patient.

Personal hygiene

In general Muslims prefer to wash in running water so a shower is preferable to a bath where possible.

Diet

Meat must be slaughtered according to the Halal ritual in which the meat is drained of blood. Halal beef, lamb and chicken are eaten but pork, carrion and blood are forbidden. Fish and eggs are allowed but must not be cooked where pork and other non-Halal meat is cooked (for example in a hospital or care home kitchen). During the month of Ramadan a Muslim must fast between sunrise and sunset. Although Muslims who are temporarily ill or who have a chronic condition may be permitted not to fast, it is important for health care staff to understand that the fasting may still compromise medical diets, tests, etc. If Halal food is not available the family should be allowed to bring food in for the patient, or a strict vegetarian diet should be offered.

Medication

Islam prohibits the consumption of alcohol so Muslims may refuse medication that contains alcohol.

Prayer

Devout Muslims will pray up to five times a day. Privacy and peace should be given to allow them to do this. Before prayer a ritual wash in running water is undertaken, in which face, hands and arms are washed in a predetermined way. If the patient is confined to bed they may need help with their preparation for prayer and a jug of water and a bowl will ensure a source of running water is available. Clothes should also be changed if they have become soiled. There is a special format for prayer that uses special hand gestures instead of whole body movements that can be carried out when the patient is confined to bed.

### Family and individual

Muslim patients tend to be visited frequently by their extended family, which can cause some difficulties with regard to the preset visiting times and 'numbers of visitor' policies which exist in most UK hospitals. Many of the visitors may also wish to be involved in the care of the patient, so they should be advised on how they may contribute. As Muslims do not generally encourage men and women to mix freely in public, Muslim patients should not be placed in mixed wards.

### Death and dying

As the person approaches death they will expect to have their family and friends around them, which can sometimes mean a considerable number of people visiting at any one time. If this happens, caring for the patient in a side room may be preferable. If members of the family are not in attendance when death occurs, health care staff should wear disposable gloves so that they do not directly touch the body. The person's head should be turned towards Mecca (usually southeast in the UK), the arms and legs straightened, eyes and mouth closed and the body covered entirely with a clean white sheet. Female bodies should be attended to by female care staff and, if at all possible, male bodies by male care staff. The remaining preparation of the body will be carried out by a member of the family, who should be contacted immediately.

## Sikhism

'Sikh' translates roughly as 'student or disciple' and originated as a reformist movement of Hinduism; its founder, Guru Nanak, attempting to combine the best features of Hinduism and Islam. Sikhs believe in one God and must live a spiritual life and develop their own individual relationship with God by dedicating their lives to doing good. Thus, while on this earth they should be truthful, gentle, kind and generous, and work towards the common good. They perceive all men as equal.

Sikhs have five 'signs' which they should wear at all times, known as the 'five Ks'.

They are:

- Kesh – uncut beard and hair;

- Kangha – wooden comb;

- Kara – a steel bracelet worn on the right wrist;

- Kirpan – a sharp knife with a double-edged blade (often now in the UK worn in the form of a badge or brooch);

- Kaccha – long underpants/trousers.

## *Considerations for practice*

### Physical examination

Generally Sikh men and women would prefer to be examined by a member of the health care staff of the same gender as themselves, and would wish to remain as covered as possible through an examination or procedure. Removal of any of the five Ks must be strictly at the agreement/permission of the patient or their family. When removed they should be treated with great care.

### Personal hygiene

Sikhs prefer to use running water for washing and thus prefer to shower rather than bathe. If a patient is unable to use a shower, a bowl and a jug of water is an acceptable alternative. Male Sikhs may also need help to remove their turban (which has to be done at least once a day). Both men and women may need help with the required regular washing, drying and combing of their hair.

### Diet

Meat that has been prepared in a ritualistic way for another religion should not be given to a Sikh. Although there are no specific rules about not eating meat, many Sikhs are vegetarian and this includes not eating fish or eggs.

### Prayer

Sikhs spend a lot of time in meditative contemplation of God. Before prayers the person will want to wash themselves and dress in clean clothes if necessary. A patient may need help to ensure this happens.

### Family and the individual

Visiting the sick is a duty of the Sikh community, so the patient may receive many visitors. Families and friends will also expect to be involved in discussions about treatment and the provision of health care. A patient may refuse treatment or care if the family does not agree with it. Sikh patients should not be placed in mixed wards

### Death and dying

If a member of the family is not available, health care staff should wear disposable gloves to avoid direct contact with the patient after death. Do not undress, wash the body or remove any of the five Ks, as that is something the family would wish to carry out themselves. Drains and other tubes can be removed. The body should then be wrapped in a clean white cloth/sheet ready for the family to care for.

## Buddhism

Buddhism is a way of life rather than an organised religion. Its focus is on personal spiritual development and the attainment of a deeper insight into the true nature of life, rather than a set of ritualistic practices. It teaches that all life is interconnected and the path to enlightenment is through the practice and development of morality, meditation and wisdom. The practice of Buddhism is extremely diverse and Buddhists from different regions will have different interpretations of the central ideas.

### *Considerations for practice*

#### Diet

Most Buddhists tend to be vegetarians.

#### Medication

Some Buddhists may refuse to accept medication that contains alcohol or animal products. Some may prefer to use other strategies, such as meditation, to relieve pain as an alternative to conventional analgesia.

#### Dying

A Buddhist who knows that they are dying will probably wish to have their family and friends with them to meditate and chant mantras as death approaches. They will need as much peace and quiet as possible to allow this to happen. After death, do not touch or move the body of a Buddhist patient until advice has been sought from an appropriate source (for example, the family, friends or the hospital chaplain).

(Clarke, 1993; Weller, 2001; Henley and Schott, 1999)

www.ethnicityonline.net

## Summary

Working with cultural diversity requires knowledge and sensitivity. Generally family members prefer to be asked about their customs and religious requirements rather than just ignoring them.

Remember that whatever cultural or religious beliefs a patient may hold, they will still have preferences and needs which are individual and personal to them alone.

> **FURTHER READING**
>
> Further reading and information on a range of religions and implications for practice in respect of health care can be obtained from the internet. Your starting point could include www.interfaith.org.uk and www.bbc.co.uk/religion.

## Legislation and policy

As a nurse there are two main pieces of legislation relating to cultural diversity that you need to be familiar with.

### The Human Rights Act (1998)

The Human Rights Act came into force in October 2000. It represents the translation of the law of the European Convention on Human Rights into UK law. This means that the UK has a legislative framework that defines standards for what each person has a right to expect with regard to fundamental human rights and freedoms. The Act covers all infringements of human rights regardless of gender, disability, ethnic identity, sexuality or class and makes it unlawful for public authorities (which includes NHS Trusts, all health authorities, private and voluntary sector contractors, social services, general practitioners, dentists, opticians and pharmacists) to act in a way that is incompatible with Convention rights, unless they are acting under legislation which makes it impossible to act differently. The Convention rights include the following:

- **Article 2: The right to life** – The state is required to make adequate provision in its laws for the protection of human life. This means they must take positive steps to protect life in all kinds of situations including admission to hospital and other health care settings. Hospitals are under a duty to take positive steps to safeguard a patient's right to life. Relevant healthcare staff may therefore need to consider the implications before refusing life-saving treatment to a patient.

- **Article 3: Freedom from torture and inhuman or degrading treatment or punishment** – This is an absolute right not to be tortured or subjected to treatment or punishment that is inhuman or degrading. How an individual's treatment is classified depends on many different factors, including their state of health. Whether or not treatment is considered degrading depends on 'whether a reasonable person of the same age or sex and health as you would have felt degraded' (DCA, 2006, p. 16).

- **Article 4: Freedom from slavery and forced or compulsory labour** – This is an absolute right not be treated like a slave or forced to perform certain kinds of labour. This might apply to a situation such as staff from overseas having their passports removed by their employers to prevent them leaving a place of work.

- **Article 5: Right to liberty, freedom and security of person** – Unless a detention is lawful, an individual cannot be deprived of their liberty for even a short period of time. Detention in this context can include detention in mental hospitals. Acceptable reasons for arrest and detention, in accordance with set procedures set down by law, include: if a person is shown to be of unsound mind, an alcoholic, a drug addict or a vagrant, or to prevent an individual spreading infectious disease.

- **Article 6: Right to a fair trial** – Every person has the right to a fair hearing, a public hearing, an independent and impartial tribunal and to a hearing within a reasonable time.

- **Article 7: Freedom from retrospective criminal law and no punishment without law** – This relates to the right to normally not be found guilty of a criminal offence that occurred at a time when the offence was not deemed a criminal act.

- **Article 8: Right to respect for private and family life, home and correspondence** – This confers the right for each person to live their own life as is reasonable within a democratic society and takes account of the freedoms and rights of others. This right can also include the right to have personal information such as official records, including medical information, kept private and confidential. This right also places restrictions on the extent to which any public authority can invade an individual's privacy about their body without their permission. It should be noted that this raises issues in procedures such as taking blood samples and the right to refuse treatment.

- **Article 9: Freedom of thought, conscience and religion** – This provides an absolute right for a person to hold the thoughts, positions of conscience or religion of their choice. This includes the right for the person to practise or demonstrate their religion in private or public (as long as it does not interfere with the rights and freedoms of others).

- **Article 10: Freedom of expression** – 'Expression' here includes personal views or opinions, speaking aloud, publication of articles or books or leaflets, television or radio broadcasting, producing works of art, communication through the internet, some forms of commercial information (DCA, 2006, p. 23).

- **Article 11: Freedom of assembly and association** – Every person has the right to 'peacefully' assemble with others.

- **Article 12: Right to marry** – this includes the right to have a family.

- **Article 14: Freedom of discrimination** – In the context of the Act, discrimination is defined as 'treating people in similar situations differently, or those in different situations in the same way, without proper justification' (DCA, 2006, p. 25). Among other issues this includes sexual orientation, age, race, colour, language, religion, disability, political or other opinion, national or social origin, association with a national minority, property, birth (for example whether born inside or outside of marriage), and marital status. Regardless of status, everyone is entitled to equal access to all the rights set out in the Act.

- **Protocol 1 of Article 2: Right to education** – No person should be denied the right to the education system and an effective education.

Articles 2, 3, 8, 9 and 14 are particularly important to nursing practice and relate to the Nursing and Midwifery Council's *Code* (2008).

---

**ACTIVITY 5.2**

Research further information regarding the Human Rights Act 1998 from www.direct.gov.uk, www.YourRights.org.uk, www.dh.gov.uk or through a general search engine such as Google. Then consider and note down the implications of Articles 2, 3, 8, 9 and 14 in relation to your practice as a student of nursing.

---

## The Equality Act 2010

The Equality Act 2010 is the law that seeks to ban unfair treatment and achieve equal opportunities in the workplace and the wider society.

The Act covers nine 'protected characteristics':

- age;
- race;
- religion or belief;
- disability;
- gender identity and gender reassignment;
- sex;
- sexual orientation;
- pregnancy and maternity;
- marriage and civil partnership.

The Equality Act sets out the different ways in which it is unlawful to treat someone, for example by direct or indirect discrimination, harassment or victimisation, and failing to make a reasonable adjustment for a disabled person.

It covers all aspects of an organisation's activities, policy and service provision and delivery, as well as employment practices. This obviously has considerable implications for your work as a nurse, both as a student and a qualified practitioner (see www.homeoffice.gov.uk).

---

**FURTHER READING**

Further reading regarding the Equality Act 2010 can be obtained from www.adviceguide.org.uk.

---

## Chapter summary

- Culture encompasses the values, beliefs, behaviour, practices and material objects that constitute a people's way of life.

- Every practitioner should seek to ensure that they provide and deliver care that meets the religious, dietary and linguistic requirements of patients while ensuring that the principle of individualised care is not compromised.

- Working with cultural diversity requires knowledge and sensitivity.

- The Human Rights Act (1998) and the Equality Act (2010) are the two main pieces of legislation relating to cultural diversity that you need to be familiar with.

## References

Andrews, M.M. & Boyle, J.S. (2007) *Transcultural Concepts in Nursing Care* (5th edition). London: Lippincott Williams and Wilkins.

Clarke, P.B. (1993) *The World's Religions*. London: Reader's Digest.

Department for Constitutional Affairs (2006) *A Guide to the Human Rights Act 1998* (3rd edition). London: DCA.

Equality Act (2010) Available from www.homeoffice.gov.uk (accessed 21 November 2012)

Geiger, J. & Davidhizar, R. (2007) *Transcultural Nursing: Assessment and Intervention* (5th edition). New York: Mosby.

Gerrish, K., Husband, C. and Mackenzie, J. (1996) *Ethnicity, the minority ethnic community and health care delivery*, in Royal College of Nursing (2006) *Transcultural Health Care Practice: An Educational Resource for Nurses and Health Care Practitioners*. Available from www.rcn.org.uk/resources/transcultural/index.php (accessed 6 January 2013)

Henley, A. & Schott, J. (1999) *Culture, Religion and Patient Care in a Multi-Ethnic Society. A Handbook for Professionals*. London: Age Concern.

Hofstede, G. & Hofstede, G.J. (2004) *Cultures and Organisations: Software of the Mind* (2nd edition). New York: McGraw Hill.

Human Rights Act (1998). Available from www.direct.gov.uk (accessed 20 November 2012)

Jirwe, M. (2008) *Cultural Competence in Nursing*. Stockholm: Karolinska Institute.

Klein, E. (1971) A *Comprehensive Etymological Dictionary of the English Language*. Amsterdam: Elsevier Scientific Publishing Co.

Leininger, M. & McFarland, M. (2002) *Transcultural Nursing* (3rd edition). New York: McGraw Hill.

Macionis, J.J. & Plummer, K. (2008) *Sociology: A Global Introduction* (4th edition). England: Pearson Education.

Nursing and Midwifery Council (2008) *The Code: Standards of Conduct, Performance and Ethics for Nurses and Midwives*. London: NMC.

Office for National Statistics (2011) *Ethnicity and National Identity in England and Wales*. Available from www.ons.gov.uk/ons/rel/census/2011-census/key-statistics-for-local-authorities-in-england-and-wales/rpt-ethnicity.html#tab-conclusions (accessed 7 January 2013)

Papadopoulos, I. (ed.) (2006) *Transcultural Health and Social Care: Development of Culturally Competent Practitioners*. Oxford: Elsevier.

Royal College of Nursing (2006) *Transcultural Health Care Practice: An Educational Resource for Nurses and Health Care Practitioners*. Available from http://www.rcn.org.uk/resources/transcultural/index.php (accessed 20 November 2012)

Wagner. A.L. (2002) *Nursing Students' Development of Caring through Creative Reflective Practice*, in Freshwater, D. (ed.) *Therapeutic Nursing:*

*Improving Patient Care through Self-awareness and Reflection*. London: Sage.

Weller, P. (ed.) (2001) *Religions in the UK: A Multi-faith Directory* (3rd edition). Derby: University of Derby.

www.ethnicityonline.net (accessed 20 November 2012)

www.diffen.com/difference/Ethnicity_vs_Race (accessed 20 November 2012)

# 06
## QUALITY ASSURANCE

The aim of this chapter is to introduce the quality assurance framework guiding health care provision in the United Kingdom (UK) and, in particular, in England.

**Learning Outcomes**

On completion of this chapter you should be able to:

- understand some of the main policies and procedures which inform and guide quality assurance in the provision of health care;

- briefly outline the concepts of clinical governance and clinical audit;

- understand issues relevant to vulnerable adults;

- understand the importance of patients' and users' views in quality assurance;

- briefly outline the key steps in the development of Integrated Care Pathways.

## Defining quality assurance

According to Marr and Giebing (1994, p. 18), at its simplest, 'quality assurance is about describing, measuring and taking action'. Within the context of health care, Lohr (1990, cited in Kelly, 2007, p. 6) defines quality assurance as 'the degree to which health services for individuals and populations increase the likelihood of desired health outcomes and are consistent with current professional knowledge'. Ransom *et al.* (2008, p. 3) suggest that for health care professionals, quality assurance is essentially about delivering 'safe, effective, efficient, timely, patient centred and equitable' care.

Quality assurance associated with the provision and delivery of health care is a relatively new idea. Before the 1980s quality assurance in the health service tended to be implicit rather than explicit. According to Dowding and Barr (2002), this was largely due to the fact that health care was felt to exist for altruistic motives rather than for profit, and these motives were not open to quality scrutiny. International influences led in 1984 to the British government launching the National Quality Campaign for both public and private industries, and within this the National Health Service (NHS) was strongly encouraged to ensure quality control systems were in place. By the 1990s specific requirements and advice on quality were being set out in government health policy. For example, The Patients' Charter (Department of Health, 1991) set down precise national standards regarding various rights and expectations for all patients. Subsequent policy and legislation, including *A First Class Service: Improving Quality in the New NHS* (Department of Health, 1998), made more specific plans for progress in improving the health service, especially in terms of effectiveness, efficiency and excellence. These plans reflected the need for clear lines of responsibility and quality management activities incorporating monitoring and continuous improvement. *A First Class Service* also identified clinical effectiveness, evidence-based practice, clinical supervision and continuing professional development activities as specific requirements for health care practitioners in support of quality assurance. Since then there have been a number of initiatives and policies, including the *Equity and Excellence: Liberating the NHS* White Paper (Department of Health, 2010a), which have identified successive governments' commitment to continually trying to improve quality of care.

# The organisation of quality assurance in UK health care

In the UK, health service quality processes can take place at both national and local level. There is no easy way to introduce you to the plethora of organisations, agencies and initiatives with a mandate to ensure quality of care provision at each of these levels. However, you need to have a basic understanding / awareness of the key agencies as you will encounter their work either directly or indirectly in your practice.

## Care Quality Commission (CQC)

The CQC began operating on April 1st 2009 as the independent regulator of all health and adult social care services in England, including those provided by the NHS, local authorities, private companies and voluntary organisations. The CQC replaced three earlier commissions, namely the Commission for Social Care Inspection, the Health Care Commission and the Mental Health

Act Commission. By law all health and adult social care providers (including the NHS) must be registered with the CQC. This also includes primary medical services and general practitioners from 2013. Without registration, providers are not allowed to operate. The Commission is funded through a combination of registration fee income and government grant-in-aid.

The role of the CQC is to ensure that the care provided in hospitals, dental surgeries (and, from April 2013, those of general practitioners (GPs)), ambulances, care homes and via services to people in their own homes and elsewhere meets the government standards of quality and safety. It also protects the interests of people detained under the Mental Health Act.

The Commission carries out its role mainly by the process of inspection. Most hospitals, care homes and domiciliary care services are inspected at least once a year and dental services biannually. There are three types of inspections that may be carried out:

- **scheduled** – these are unannounced inspections that focus on a minimum of five of the government's standards, and are tailored to the type of care provided by the service;

- **responsive** – unannounced inspections that respond to concerns about poor care being provided;

- **themed** – inspections that focus on specific standards of care or care services.

An important part of the Commission's work is collecting data from service users' experiences of care services. In some cases it involves patients and their carers directly in working alongside its inspectors to give an expert user view of services.

It also makes use of all informal and formal information and data to monitor what is happening inside health and social care systems, as well as across both health and social care, in order to identify where a pattern of incidents indicates that something untoward may be happening.

If a provider is not meeting the government standards of quality and safety then the Commission has a range of legal powers and duties to enforce the appropriate standards. These include:

- issuing a warning notice requiring improvements within a set period of time;

- restricting the services the provider can offer;

- stopping admission to the care service;

- issuing fixed penalty notices, suspending or cancelling the service's registration;

- prosecution.

In order to enforce the standards the Commission is able, depending on the circumstances, to liaise with other agencies including local authorities, regulatory bodies (for example, Monitor, the independent regulator of foundation trusts – see below), Directors of Adult Social Services and the police (www.nhs.uk; www.cqc.org.uk).

The Care Quality Commission does not have a remit in Scotland or Northern Ireland. These each have their own similar regulatory bodies.

## Monitor

Formerly, the main role of Monitor was as the independent regulator of Foundation Trusts. Following the introduction of the Health and Social Care Act 2012, Monitor has become the regulator for all providers of NHS funded services in England. Under the Act, all providers will be required (unless exempt under specific regulations made by the Secretary of State for Health) to hold a Monitor licence.

The licence will set out a range of conditions that providers must meet and it will be used to carry out Monitor's main duties, that is, to protect and promote the interests of people who use health care services. The aim is to achieve this by promoting provision of services that are economic, efficient and effective, and which maintain or improve the quality of services.

Monitor will have a range of enforcement powers that allow action to be taken in cases of breach of licence.

N.B. The proposed requirement to hold a licence would not replace any requirement for providers to be registered with the Care Quality Commission. The CQC and Monitor have established a framework for working together across the services.

(www.monitor-nhsft.gov.uk)

## The Health and Safety Executive (HSE)

The HSE is the national independent regulator for health and safety in the workplace. This includes private or publicly owned health and social care settings throughout the UK. The HSE does not normally investigate issues of clinical judgement or matters that relate to the quality of care provided. However, it does take the lead on employee health and safety and may also deal with non-clinical risks to patients (for example trips, falls, scalding, electrical safety, etc.). It also deals with aspects of risk that apply to both staff and patients (for example manual handling). In order to fulfil its role the HSE works in partnership with co-regulators in local authorities to inspect, investigate and where necessary take enforcement action.

(www.hse.gov.uk)

## NHS complaints procedure

This complaints procedure covers complaints made by a patient or person about any matter connected with the provision of NHS services by NHS organisations or primary care practitioners (GPs, dentists, opticians and pharmacists). The procedure also covers services provided overseas and by the private sector where the NHS has paid for them. If an individual is dissatisfied with the treatment or service they have received from the NHS they are entitled to make a complaint, have it considered, and receive a response from the NHS organisation or primary care practitioner concerned. The complaint can also be made by someone acting on behalf of the patient or person with their consent. The complaint must normally be made within 12 months of the event or within 12 months of becoming aware that the person has something to complain about. These time limits can be waived if there is good reason to do so.

Under the NHS Constitution an individual making a complaint has the right to:

- have their complaint dealt with efficiently, and properly investigated;

- know the outcome of any investigation into their complaint;

- take the complaint to the Independent Parliamentary and Health Service Ombudsman if they are not satisfied with the way the NHS has dealt with the complaint;

- make a claim for a judicial review if they think they have been directly affected by an unlawful act or decision of an NHS body;

- receive compensation if they have been harmed.

(Department of Health, 2010b, p. 8)

The first stage of the procedure is known as 'local resolution', with the complaint, in the first instance, being made to the organisation or primary care practitioner who provided the services. Initially this may be by voicing concerns to a member of staff or the Patient Advice and Liaison Service (PALS). However, if the individual wishes to make the complaint more formal, they can do so either orally or in writing (including email) to the organisation's complaints manager. If the individual is not satisfied with the response to their complaint they can request or agree to an 'independent review' of their case through the Health Service Ombudsman. This is an independent body set up to investigate complaints about health services and promote improvements of health care as a result. Financial compensation, legal action and professional misconduct are not dealt with through this process.

(www.nhs.uk; www.pals.nhs)

---

**FURTHER READING**

Further information on monitoring and promoting improvement of quality of health care in Wales, Scotland and Northern Ireland can be obtained from: www.hiw.org.uk, www.healthcareimprovementscotland.org and www.dhsspsni.gov.uk, respectively.

---

## Local clinical level

Quality assurance at local level covers a variety of activities including clinical audit, patients' and users' views and patient advisory services. Further issues such as the Protection of Vulnerable Adults, Integrated Care Pathways and the *Essence of Care* (Department of Health, 2010c) initiative can also be included here.

### Clinical governance

Clinical governance is a very broad concept. Introduced in 1998, it placed quality at the centre of proposed NHS reforms by building on earlier efforts to audit, monitor and improve practice. The Department of Health defined it as:

> a framework through which organizations are accountable for continuously improving the quality of their services and safeguarding

high standards of care by creating an environment in which excellence in clinical care will flourish.

(Department of Health, 1998, p. 33)

Som (2004) sought to encompass the complexity of the contributing factors and organisation-wide implications for continuous quality improvement, stating that:

> Clinical governance is defined as a governance system for healthcare organisations that promotes an integrated approach towards management of inputs, structures and processes to improve the outcome of health-care service delivery where health staff work in an environment of greater accountability for clinical quality.

(Som, 2004, p. 89)

Covering the organisation's systems and processes for monitoring and improving services, the key elements of clinical governance include:

- Strong leadership and accountability;

- Patient, public, carer consultation and involvement;

- Clinical effectiveness and commitment to quality;

- Clinical audit

- Education, training and continuous professional development;

- Research and development;

- Clinical risk management;

- Staff management and performance;

- Use of information about patients' experiences, outcomes and processes.

All of the key elements are of equal value and importance and all are interrelated.

In essence, clinical governance is perceived as being about ensuring safe, high quality care from those involved in a patient's journey, while ensuring the patient remains the main focus and priority.

**FURTHER READING**

Further information on clinical governance can be accessed from: www.dh.gov.
uk/en/Publicationsandstatistics/Lettersandcirculars/Healthservicecirculars/
DH_4004883. This document provides succinct but relatively comprehensive
coverage of the government's aims and policy principles and implementation of
clinical governance in the NHS.

**ACTIVITY 6.1**

Access the RCN website (www.rcn.org.uk) and type 'clinical governance' in the
search box. This RCN web resource aims to help nurses become more involved
with local and national quality improvement projects.

### Clinical audit

Clinical audit is an essential and integral part of clinical governance at
local level. It is a quality improvement process that was introduced by the
1989 White Paper *Working for Patients*. The Department of Health in 1989
defined clinical audit as:

> ... the systematic and critical analysis of the quality of clinical care,
> including the procedures used for diagnosis, treatment and care, the
> associated use of resources and the resulting outcome and quality of
> life for the patient.
>
> (Department of Health, 1989)

The National Institute for Health and Clinical Excellence describes it as:

> ...a quality improvement process that seeks to improve the patient
> care and outcomes through systematic review of the care against
> explicit criteria and implementation of change.
>
> (NICE, 2002, p. 1)

Essentially, clinical audit is about clinical effectiveness and quality
improvement and is now a key component of the clinical governance
framework and well established both within the NHS and the independent sector.

The key elements of clinical audit are:

- setting standards / criteria for a chosen area / topic;

- measuring current practice;

- comparing the results with the standards / criteria set;

- changing practice if required;

- re-auditing to ensure quality practice has been maintained or practice has improved.

Put together, these elements are usually referred to as the 'audit cycle'.

The fundamental principles associated with clinical audit are that it should:

- be professionally led;

- be viewed as an educational process;

- be a routine part of clinical practice;

- be based on the setting of standards;

- generate results based on the setting of standards;

- generate results that can be used to improve outcome of quality care;

- involve management in both the process and outcome of audit;

- be confidential at the individual patient / clinician level;

- be informed by the views of patients / clients.

(NHS Executive, 1994; Burgess, 2010)

### Patients' and users' views

Since the early 2000s there has been a clear move by the government towards a culture of regularly involving and consulting patients and the public in decision-making and service improvement. In 2003 the Health and Social Care Act placed a duty on the NHS to engage actively with community and service users. In October 2008 this was taken a stage further when the government published the Local Government and Public Health Act. This Act contained new duties for health organisations to reinforce and improve the way the NHS pays attention to and utilises the views of the public to improve local health services.

Healthwatch

The Health and Social Care Act 2012 provides for the establishment of Healthwatch England as a statutory committee of the Care Quality Commission. Healthwatch England is part of a Healthwatch network which seeks to give a more powerful voice, both locally and nationally, to the key issues that affect people who use health and social care services.

Views from all sections of the community are sought and it functions at two levels:

- Healthwatch England – works at a national level

  - providing leadership, support and advice to local Healthwatch organisations;

  - gathering and analysing information provided by local Healthwatch organisations;

  - ensuring the views of people who use health and social care services are relayed to the Secretary of State, the Care Quality Commission, the NHS Commissioning Board, Monitor and all local authorities in England.

- Local Healthwatch Organisations will

  - cover every local authority in England;

  - have the power to enter and view services;

  - be able to influence how services are set up and commissioned by having a seat on the local health and wellbeing board;

  - produce reports which may influence the way services are both designed and delivered;

  - provide information, advice and support about local services;

  - provide information and recommendations to Healthwatch England and the Care Quality Commission;

  - be based in and funded by Local Authorities;

  - also encompass the functions currently / previously carried out by Local Involvement Networks (LINKs).

    (www.healthwatch.co.uk; www.dh.gov)

The Patient Advice and Liaison Service (PALS)

Established throughout the NHS, this service offers confidential support and advice directly to service users, families and carers if they have a perceived cause for complaint or concern. Although not part of the complaints procedure itself, the service liaises with staff, managers and, where appropriate, other relevant organisations, to negotiate informally and encourage fast solution of the problem or concern. The core functions of PALS are to:

- be identifiable and accessible to patients, their carers, friends and families;

- provide on the spot help in every Trust with the power to negotiate immediate solutions or speedy resolution of problems;

- act as a gateway to appropriate independent advice and advocacy support from local and national sources;

- provide accurate information to patients, carers and families, about the Trust's services, and about other health-related issues;

- act as a catalyst for change and improvement by providing the Trust with information and feedback on problems arising and gaps in services;

- operate within a local network with other PALS in their area and work across organisational boundaries;

- support staff at all levels within the Trust to develop a responsive culture.

(www.pals.nhs.uk)

## Further issues

### Protection of vulnerable adults

A vulnerable adult is defined broadly as:

> ...a person who is or may be in need of community care services by reason of mental or other disabilities, age or illness; and who is or may be unable to take care of him or herself, or unable to protect him or herself against significant harm or exploitation.

(Department of Health, 2000)

Following a number of high profile serious incidents involving vulnerable adults, the Department of Health published *No Secrets: Guidance on Developing and Implementing Multi-agency Policies and Procedures to Protect*

*Vulnerable Adults from Abuse* (2000). This document provides guidance on actions to be taken within health and social care regarding the appropriate protection and support of vulnerable adults. The aim of the guidance has been to construct a framework in which all relevant agencies are required to work together to ensure strong and coherent policies and procedures are in place, and implemented locally for the protection of vulnerable adults who are at risk of abuse. Abuse in this context is defined by the Department of Health (2000, p. 9) as 'a violation of an individual's human and civil rights by another person or persons'.

The abuse may be a single or repeated act, may occur in any relationship and may result in serious harm to, or exploitation of, the person subjected to it. The main forms of abuse can be identified as:

- **physical abuse** (includes misuse of medication and restraint);

- **sexual abuse**;

- **psychological abuse** (includes verbal abuse, controlling and withdrawal from services or supportive networks);

- **financial / material abuse** (includes theft, fraud and misuse or misappropriation of possessions);

- **neglect and acts of omission** (includes ignoring medical or physical care needs and withholding necessities of life such as medication and adequate nutrition);

- **discriminatory abuse** (includes racist, sexist and ageist abuse and harassment).

A further form of abuse, referring specifically to neglect and poor professional practice, is often referred to as 'institutional abuse'. This ranges from an isolated event of poor or unsatisfactory professional practice through to ongoing ill treatment or gross misconduct.

The NMC defines abuse within the registrant–client relationship as 'the result of the misuse of power or a betrayal of trust, respect or intimacy between the registrant and the client, which the registrant should know would cause physical or emotional harm to the client' (NMC, 2007, p. 2). Its guidance, which defines the standards of conduct within the registrant / client / patient relationship, identifies zero tolerance of abuse as the only philosophy consistent with protecting the public. It stresses that registrants have a responsibility to ensure that they safeguard the interests of their clients at all times and to protect patients / clients from all forms of abuse. If, in the course of their professional practice, registrants suspect or believe that a client is being, or has been abused, they must report this as soon as practical to a person of appropriate authority. This zero tolerance of abuse is also expected from students of nursing.

In 2010 the NMC published the guidelines *Raising and Escalating Concerns*. The purpose of the guidance is to 'establish principles for best practice in the raising and escalating of concerns (also known as whistleblowing). It explains the process you should follow when raising concerns, provides information about legislation in this area and indicates where you can access confidential support and advice' (NMC, 2010, p. 1).

---

## ACTIVITY 6.2

You should access, read and keep a copy of the guidelines *Raising and Escalating Concerns: Guidance for Nurses and Midwives* from www.nmc-uk.org. Other documents that you may find useful include *Every Child Matters* (Department of Education, 2003) and *What to do if you're Worried a Child is Being Abused* (Department for Education and Skills, 2006). Both are available from www.education.gov.uk.

---

### *Disclosure and Barring Service (DBS)*

Disclosure

Under the 2012 Protection of Freedom Act, and in order to provide a more seamless service, the Independent Safeguarding Authority and the Criminal Records Bureau merged to form the Disclosure and Barring Service (DBS).

The DBS searches police records and, where relevant, barred list information and then issues a DBS certificate to an applicant and employer. The checking service currently offers two levels of DBS check – standard and enhanced.

Referrals

Part of the role of the DBS is to help prevent unsuitable people from working with vulnerable groups, including children. Referrals are made to the DBS when an employer or an organisation has a concern that a person has caused harm or poses a future risk of harm to vulnerable groups. A wide range of employers and organisations are required or empowered to make referrals and these include Trusts, the General Medical Council and the Nursing and Midwifery Council.

Barring

The Barred Lists are a database of people barred from working with children or vulnerable adults. These two lists provide a record of:

- individuals who will not be permitted to work in regulated activity with children and/or vulnerable adults;

- individuals who can only work with children and/or vulnerable adults in controlled activities with safeguards.

The DBS considers a range of information from the police and referrals from employers, regulatory bodies and other agencies as part of a specifically developed decision-making process on whether to include a person on a list.

The DBS will not remove a bar unless it is satisfied that the individual does not pose a risk of harm to children or vulnerable adults.

(www.homeoffice.gov.uk; www.newham.gov.uk)

## FURTHER READING

Further information related to the *No Secrets: Guidance on Developing and Implementing Multi-agency Policies and Procedures to Protect Vulnerable Adults from Abuse* (Department of Health, 2000) document and the protection of vulnerable adults can be accessed from www.dh.gov.uk by following the policy guidance/health and social care links.

For current information on the new vetting and barring scheme go to www.homeoffice.gov.uk or www.dh.gov.uk.

For information for Wales go to www.new.wales.gov.uk, for Scotland www.scotland.gov.uk and for Northern Ireland go to www.northernireland.gov.uk.

## *Integrated Care Pathways (ICP)*

Integrated Care Pathways may also be known as clinical pathways, multi-disciplinary pathways of care, pathways of care, care maps, collaborative care pathways and care profiles. Integrated Care Pathways can be defined as 'anticipated care placed in an appropriate time frame, written and agreed by a multidisciplinary team' (Davis, 2005).

The main feature of ICPs is that they are multidisciplinary, locally agreed, evidence-based plans and records of care that are patient-focused and that attempt to view the provision of care in terms of the 'patient's journey'. They detail decisions to be made and the care to be provided for a given patient or group for a given condition in a step-wise sequence and within a given timescale. They also incorporate intermediate and long-term outcome criteria and a variance record which allows deviations from the planned care to be documented and analysed. Variations from the pathway may occur as clinical judgement is exercised to meet the needs of the individual patient.

According to Middleton *et al.* (2001) initially the development of such pathways concentrated on specific surgical conditions such as total hip replacements and the more 'predictable' medical conditions such as stroke or acute myocardial infarction, which generally offered a definable sequence of events. However, ICPs are increasingly being utilised for less predictable conditions. Because they are locally agreed and developed it is not possible to provide an overall list of the conditions for which an ICP might be introduced; however, examples include:

- care of the elderly: acute admission;

- acute pneumonia;

- inflammatory bowel disease;

- asthma;

- prostatectomy;

- mastectomy;

- aortic valve replacement.

A considerable number of benefits are identified in the literature with regard to the use of integrated care pathways; these include the following:

- they encourage the translation of national guidelines into local protocols and their subsequent application to clinical practice;

- they result in more complete and accessible data collection for audit and encourage changes in practice;

- they encourage multidisciplinary communication and care planning;

- they promote more patient-focused care and improve patient information by letting the patient see what is planned and what progress is expected;

- they enable new staff to learn quickly the key interventions for specific conditions and to appreciate likely variations;

- they facilitate multidisciplinary audit and prompt incorporation of improvements in the care into routine practice;

- they support the introduction of evidence-based practice and use of clinical guidelines;

- they can support continuity and co-ordination of care across different clinical disciplines and sectors;

- they provide explicit and well-defined standards for care;

- they help reduce variations in patient care (by promoting standardisation) and improve clinical outcomes;

- they help improve and even reduce patient documentation by streamlining and combining multidisciplinary documentation;

- they disseminate accepted standards of care;

- they provide all carers with information on a client's progress and status;

- they make explicit the standards of care against which actual care can be judged;

- patients are able to receive realistic expectations about their conditions and their expected progress;

- full compliance with ICPs meets the NMC standards for clinical record keeping.

The key steps in developing an integrated care pathway are:

- An important area of practice is selected.

- A multidisciplinary team is formed.

- Current clinical evidence for care of the patient group is compared with established clinical guidelines in all areas of practice.

- The integrated care pathway is developed (which specifies elements of care detailed in local protocols, the sequence of events and expected patient progress over time).

- The ICP is piloted and the outcomes reviewed.

- If necessary the pathway is revised.

- The ICP is implemented.

- Regular analysis of any variants from the pathway is undertaken (for example, investigating the reasons why practice was different from that recommended in the ICP).

As a student nurse your involvement in ICPs may include:

- using one in practice;

- developing a pathway for a specific condition;

- evaluating a pathway that has already been developed;

- teaching other members of staff about their use.

(Middleton *et al.*, 2001; Fisher and McMillan, 2004; www.csp.org.uk; www.medsci.ox.ac.uk; www.wales.nhs.uk; www.rcn.org.uk; www.openclinical.org/clinicalpathways.html)

---

**ACTIVITY 6.3**

Access further information regarding the development and implementation of ICPs using a general search engine such as Google. You should find the sample documentation available on many of the sites useful for future practice.

---

## *Essence of Care*

The original *Essence of Care* benchmarks were developed in 2001. They are a tool to help health care practitioners take a patient-focused and structured approach to sharing and comparing practice. They were also designed to support measures to improve quality, and to contribute to clinical governance within organisations. *Essence of Care* focuses on what might be described as the fundamental and essential aspects of care and it seeks to enable health care personnel to work with patients to identify best practice and to develop action plans to improve care.

The updated *Essence of Care 2010* (Department of Health, 2010c) supports and reflects a number of the themes in *Equity and Excellence: Liberating the NHS* (Department of Health, 2010a) and provides a set of benchmarks to encourage best practice in delivering the fundamentals of care and improving the experiences of people who use services.

It can be used by individuals, teams, directorates, and within and across organisations of all sizes. It can also be used locally or strategically, or ideally, both.

## Benchmarking tools

In the context of the document *Essence of Care 2010* (Department of Health, 2010c) a benchmark is 'a standard of best practice and care by which current practice and care is assessed or measured' (Department of Health, 2010c, p. 9).

Following from this benchmarking is 'a systematic process in which current practice and care are compared to, and amended to attain, best practice and care' (Department of Health, 2010c, p. 9).

The *Essence of Care 2010* benchmarks comprise:

• an overall person-focused outcome that expresses what people and carers want from care in a particular area of practice;

• definitions of terms as appropriate;

• general indicators, or goals, for best practice;

• a number of factors, or topics, that need to be considered in order to achieve the overall person-focused outcome.

Each factor consists of:

• a person-focused statement of best practice and care which is placed at the extreme right of the continuum;

• a statement of poor practice and care which is placed at the extreme left of the continuum;

• indicators, or goals, identified by people, carers, association representatives and staff that support the attainment of best practice and care.

Patients, carers and professionals worked together to agree and describe person-focused outcomes, specific factors and indicators within the benchmarks in twelve areas of care:

- personal hygiene;

- respect and dignity;

- food and nutrition;

- self care;

- safety;

- record keeping;

- prevention and management of pain;

- prevention and management of pressure ulcers;

- bladder, bowel and continence care;

- communication (between patients, carers and health care personnel);

- promoting health and wellbeing;

- care environment.

It should be recognised that all sets of benchmarks are interrelated (Department of Health, 2010c).

### Using clinical benchmarks

*Essence of Care 2010* benchmarking is a systematic process in which the current practice of health and social care organisations, teams or individual staff is compared to, and amended to attain, best practice and care. Changes and improvements focus on the indicators, or goals, within the factors, since these are the items that people, carers and staff believe are important for achieving best practice and care.

Briefly the steps involved are:

**Step one:** establish priorities for improving practice and care within the environment or organisation.

**Step two:** establish and agree best (evidence-based) practice and care for people within the organisation.

**Step three:** ascertain current practice and care.

**Step four:** compare the differences, and identify the gaps and barriers between, current and best practice and care and identify achievements.

**Step five:** develop a plan of what goals need to be met to achieve best practice and care; that is, working out what needs to be done and how.

**Step six:** implement the plan (that is, change things, for example, activity, perspective, approach, culture, education and training, environment, etc.) to meet the goals.

**Step seven:** evaluate practice and care by assessing and measuring whether goals have been met.

**Step eight:** establish improved practice and care across a team or organisation(s).

**Step nine:** establish priorities and further goals to continuously improve quality of practice and care; that is, go through the steps again.

The benchmarks are relevant to all health and social care settings. Therefore, the *Essence of Care* is presented in a generic format in order that it can be used in, for example, primary, secondary and tertiary settings and with all patient and/or carer groups, such as in paediatric care, mental health, cancer care, surgery and medicine (Department of Health, 2010c).

---

### ACTIVITY 6.4

It is very important that you understand *Essence of Care* as you will no doubt be involved at some point in its implementation, whilst working both as a student of nursing and as a qualified practitioner. Access and read the full document at www.dh.gov.uk.

---

## Chapter summary

- Quality assurance is essentially about delivering safe, effective, efficient, timely, patient-centred and equitable care.

- In the UK health service quality processes can take place at both national and local level.

- At local level quality assurance covers a variety of activities including clinical governance, clinical audit, patients' and users' views and patient advisory services.

- The protection of vulnerable adults, integrated care pathways and the *Essence of Care* initiatives can also be included in the processes.

# References

Burgess, R. (ed.) (2010) *New Principles of Best Practice in Clinical Audit* (2nd edition). Abingdon: Radcliffe Publishing.

Davis, N. (ed.) (2005) *Integrated Care Pathways – a Guide to Good Practice.* Wales: National Leadership and Innovation Agency for Healthcare. Available from www.wales.nhs.uk/sitesplus/documents/829/ integratedcarepathways.pdf (accessed 20 November 2012)

Department for Education and Skills (2006) *What to do if you're Worried a Child is Being Abused.* London: DfES Publications.

Department of Education (2003) *Every Child Matters.* London: HMSO.

Department of Health (1989) *Working for Patients.* London: HMSO.

Department of Health (1991) *The Patient's Charter.* London: HMSO.

Department of Health (1998) *A First Class Service – Improving Quality in the New NHS.* London: Department of Health.

Department of Health (2000) *No Secrets: Guidance on Developing and Implementing Multi-agency Policies and Procedures to Protect Vulnerable Adults from Abuse.* London: Department of Health.

Department of Health (2003) The Health and Social Care Act. London: Department of Health.

Department of Health (2007) Mental Health Act. London: Department of Health.

Department of Health (2008) Local Government and Public Health Act. London: Department of Health.

Department of Health (2010a) *Equity and Excellence: Liberating the NHS.* London: Department of Health.

Department of Health (2010b) *The NHS Constitution: the NHS Belongs to us*. London: Department of Health.

Department of Health (2010c) *Essence of Care*. London: Department of Health.

Department of Health (2012a) The Health and Social Care Act 2012. London: Department of Health.

Department of Health (2012b) Protection of Freedom Act. London: Department of Health.

Dowding, L. & Barr, J. (2002) *Managing in Healthcare*. Harlow: Pearson Education.

Fisher, A. & McMillan, R. (2004) *Integrated Care Pathways for Day Surgery Patients: Guidelines for the Development, Implementation and Monitoring of Care Pathways*. Available from www.daysurgeryuk. net/bads/joomla/files/Handbooks/IntegratedCarePathways.pdf (accessed 20 November 2012)

Kelly, D.L. (2007) *Applying Quality Management in Healthcare. A Systems Approach* (2nd edition). Chicago: Health Administration Press.

Marr, H. & Giebing, H. (1994) *Quality Assurance in Nursing: Concepts, Methods and Case Studies*. Oxford: Campion Press.

Middleton, S., Barnett, J. & Reeves, D. (2001) *What is an Integrated Care Pathway?* Hayward Medical Communications. Available from www.medicine.ox.ac.uk/bandolier/painres/download/whatis/ what_is_an_icp.pdf (accessed 14 January 2013)

National Institute for Clinical Excellence (2002) *Principles for Best Practice in Clinical audit*. Oxford: Radcliffe Medical Press.

NHS Executive (1994) *The Evolution of Clinical Audit*. London: HMSO.

Nursing and Midwifery Council (2007) Registrant / client Relationships and the Prevention of Abuse. Available from www.nmc-org.uk (accessed 20 November 2012)

Nursing and Midwifery Council (2010) *Raising and Escalating Concerns. Guidance for Nurses and Midwives*. Available from www.nmc-uk.org/ Documents/Raising-and-Escalating-Concerns/Raising-and-escalating-concerns-guidance-A5.pdf (accessed 20 November 2012)

Ransom, E.R., Joshi, M.S., Nash, D.B. & Ransom, S.B. (eds) (2008) *The Healthcare Quality Book: Vision, Strategy and Tools*. Chicago: Health Administration Press.

Som, C.W. (2004) Clinical governance: A fresh look at its definition. *Clinical Governance: An International Journal*, **9(2)**: 87–89.

www.pals.nhs.uk (accessed 14 January 2013)

www.csp.org.uk (accessed 20 November 2012)

www.cqc.org.uk/public (accessed 20 November 2012)

www.monitor-nhsft.gov.uk (accessed 20 November 2012)

www.nhs.uk/NHSEngland/thenhs/healthregulators/Pages/carequalitycommission.aspx (accessed 13 January 2013)

www.nhs.uk./choiceinthenhs/rightsandpledges/complaints/pages/nhscomplaints.aspx (accessed 20 November 2012)

www.hse.gov.uk/healthservices/arrangements.htm (accessed 20 November 2012)

www.nhs.uk/NHSEngland/links/yourrights/Pages/whylink.aspx (accessed 20 November 2012)

www.homeoffice.gov.uk (accessed 20 November 2012)

www.medicine.ox.ac.uk/bandolier/booth/glossary/icp.html (accessed 20 November 2012)

www.wales.nhs.uk/sitesplus/documents/829/integratedcarepathways.pdf (accessed 14 January 2013)

www.rcn.org.uk/development/practice/perioperative_fasting/good_practice/service_improvement_tools/care_pathways (accessed 14 Jan 2013)

www.healthwatch.co.uk/about-us (accessed 21 February 2013)

www.dh.gov.uk/health/files/2012/06/B3.-Factsheet-Greater-voice-for-patients-300512.pdf (accessed 21 February 2013)

www.homeoffice.gov.uk/crime/vetting-barring-scheme (accessed 21 February 2013)

www.newham.gov.uk/NR/rdonlyres/885EB273-9517-446D-882B-D197D64CC3A3/0/FactSheet4ISABarringScheme.pdf (accessed 21 February 2013)

# 07
# EVIDENCE-BASED PRACTICE

The aim of this chapter is to remind you about the importance of respecting research and evidence-based practice within your nursing role, both as a student and when you register with the NMC.

| Learning Outcomes | • understand the concept of evidence-based practice; |
| --- | --- |
| On completion of this chapter you should be able to: | • appreciate the need to consider the evidence base when carrying out nursing care, and the challenges involved. |

## Introduction

Historically nursing and, specifically, clinical procedures, have been based on rituals rather than research (Dougherty and Lister, 2011), but over the last few decades the term 'evidence-based practice' has become common parlance within the nursing profession. Many authors have proffered definitions as to what evidence-based practice involves: Ingersoll (2000, p. 152) suggests that 'evidence-based nursing practice is the conscientious, explicit and judicious use of theory-derived, research-based information in making decisions about care delivery to individuals or groups of patients with consideration of individual needs and preferences'. Aveyard and Sharp (2009, p. 4) simplify this by saying it '...is practice that is supported by a clear, up-to-date rationale, taking into account the patient/client's preferences and using your own judgement'. Dawes et al. (2005) believe evidence-based practice ensures that decisions on patient management are made using evidence that has been critically appraised and presented in understandable terms rather than research jargon. Finally, Hamer and Collinson (2005, p. 6) add that the 'ultimate goal of evidence-based

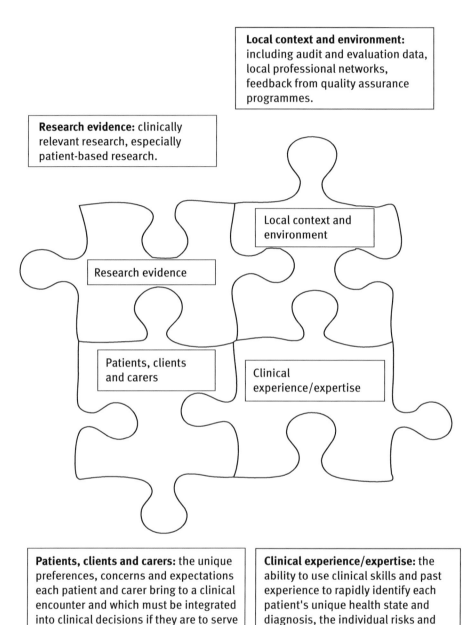

Figure 7.1 – Components of evidence-based practice (adapted from Rycroft-Malone et al., 2004)

practice is to support the practitioner in their decision making in order to eliminate the use of ineffective, inappropriate, too expensive and potentially dangerous practices'.

Notwithstanding the above definitions, the central tenet of evidence-based practice is that practitioners combine their clinical or practice expertise and their knowledge of the client or patient with the high quality evidence from research (Sackett *et al.*, 1996). Lindsay (2007) emphasises that practice requires students not only to perform skilfully but also to support their actions by referring to evidence. It is therefore an opportunity to bridge the gap between research on the one hand, and practice on the other.

*Figure 7.1* gives an example of the relationship between the three components of evidence-based practice (from Rycroft-Malone *et al.*, 2004).

## Evidence-based practice in nursing

In undertaking professional roles nurses need to understand how information derived from research is turned into 'evidence' and thus informs practice. The NMC (NMC, 2008, clause 35) clearly identifies that nurses have a responsibility to 'deliver care based on the best available evidence or best practice'. The Department of Health points out that the expectations of patients can be considered as a driver for nursing practice – 'patients are more knowledgeable and expect to be treated as partners and equals, and have to have choices and opinions available to them' (Department of Health, 2006, p. 6).

Evidence-based practice in nursing has its roots in the evidence-based medicine movement but, in nursing, definitions of the term give prominence to the patients' views of effectiveness. The RCN (1996a) emphasises this by saying:

> Evidence-based health care is rooted in the best scientific evidence and takes into account patients' views of effectiveness and clinical expertise in order to promote clinically effective services. This is essential in ensuring that health care practitioners do the things that work and are acceptable to patients, and do not do the things which don't work.
>
> (RCN, 1996a, cited in McClarey and Duff, 1997, p. 31)

This is endorsed by NHS Scotland (2005), who go further when saying that nurses must show they are doing the right thing, in the right way, at the right time, in the right place, and get the right result. They add that it includes thinking critically about what you do, questioning whether it is having the desired result, and making a change to practice; all based on evidence of what is effective in order to improve patient care and experience.

Williamson *et al.* (2008) call these factors the 'Six Rs of clinical effectiveness', as illustrated in *Figure 7.2*.

| The right person | Was the person delivering the care competent, with the right skills and knowledge? |
|---|---|
| The right thing | Was there evidence to support the intervention, and was the patient agreeable? |
| The right way | Was an intervention used correctly, with correct skills and competence, or meet national guidelines and priorities? |
| The right place | Could the patient have been treated at home, or was there a more appropriate place based on specialist equipment or staff? |
| The right time | Was the intervention timely – would it have been more effective without a six-month wait? |
| The right result | Did it do what was intended? |

*Figure 7.2 – Six Rs of clinical effectiveness (Williamson* et al.*, 2008, adapted from Bury and Mead, 1998)*

Such statements by the RCN and others clearly highlight the importance of evidence-based practice in nursing. Parahoo (2006) points out that nurses represent the largest group of health care professionals throughout the world and spend considerably more time with patients than any other health professional group. Therefore, as a profession, nursing must build its body of knowledge on solid ground. However, Craig and Smyth (2007) issue a note of caution to this – the huge range of settings and people that nurses work with can be detrimental to implementing evidence-based practice; the settings in which nurses work are so varied that research cannot possibly be relevant to all. So, what is the right thing, and what are the choices available? Craig and Smyth (2007) believe that because of the range of settings and people with which nurses work, the concept of evidence-based practice is particularly challenging for them.

Lindsay (2007, p. 4) outlines what he considers the most important reasons for practice to be based on evidence as:

- the public no longer trusts health and social care professionals to do what is best;

- professionals are conscious of the risk of being sued and want clear evidence for their practices;

- emerging health and social care professions want to create their own evidence for their roles;

- governments demand clear evidence before funding expensive new treatments or care strategies.

The NMC further endorses the concept of evidence-based practice as a means of improving the quality of care. In their *Standards for Pre-registration Nursing Education* (2010) they state that in order to offer holistic care and a range of treatment options, a newly registered nurse must make care person-centred and use evidence-based judgements and decisions to ensure high quality care. Nurses should:

- question;

- critically appraise evidence;

- take into account ethical considerations;

- take into account the individual preferences of the person receiving care;

- use evidence to support arguments.

There are many reasons why using evidence-based practice in nursing is important, and the list below does not cover them all but is a starting point:

- establishes justifiable, defensible reasons for nursing actions;

- increases cost-effective practice;

- enhances clinical effectiveness;

- is a basis for assuring quality care delivery (clinical governance);

- improves the patient's experience;

- provides evidence of what does not work;

- provides evidence to support resource allocation;

- supports managing risk;

- encourages academic and professional development.

## Carrying out evidence-based practice

Several authors (Williamson *et al.*, 2008; Offredy, 2006; Sackett *et al.*, 2000) suggest a sequence of events that has to take place before information can be considered 'evidence-based'. This is summarised in *Figure 7.3*.

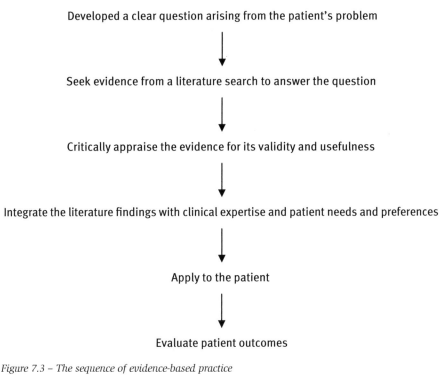

Developed a clear question arising from the patient's problem

Seek evidence from a literature search to answer the question

Critically appraise the evidence for its validity and usefulness

Integrate the literature findings with clinical expertise and patient needs and preferences

Apply to the patient

Evaluate patient outcomes

*Figure 7.3 – The sequence of evidence-based practice*

### What is evidence?

In the past, proponents of evidence-based practice have focused on research derived from quantitative methods (data collected in the form of numbers), as they were deemed the only studies worth considering. There was little or no recognition of research gathered by qualitative means (data collected in the form of words) (Ingersoll, 2000). Dougherty and Lister (2011) believe this was worrying when, within nursing, qualitative research is the prevalent design used. However, this is changing as, increasingly, evidence is recognised as coming from many different areas (as shown in *Figure 7.1*), with the proviso that it has been subjected to testing and been found credible (Higgs *et al.*, 2008).

Credibility is key in evidence-based practice but there is little consensus about how evidence is assessed before it is used to inform practice, mainly because making such judgements about evidence is complex and difficult to achieve (Dougherty and Lister, 2011). In some instances government bodies have developed nationally accepted guidelines as a result of expert researchers undertaking research trials – examples of these are the NICE guidelines and National Service Frameworks (NSFs), which were developed to achieve consistent clinical standards across the NHS. In other instances, hospitals have created their own nursing guidelines, where procedures are regularly reviewed and updated. Examples of these include the Royal Marsden Hospital's *Clinical Nursing Procedures* (Dougherty and Lister, 2011) and the Liverpool care pathway for the dying patient (www.liv.ac.uk/mcpcil/ liverpool-care-pathway, 2008). These are then published, thereby enabling other healthcare professionals and patients to benefit from the work.

## ACTIVITY 7.1

Where might you obtain information about specific evidence-based practice required to deliver high quality nursing care? Make a list of the resources available to nurses.

### Critical awareness

Society's health care needs are constantly changing. This requires nurses to keep their knowledge up to date if they are to provide the best possible care to patients. Equally, nurses need to challenge everyday practices to ensure they are safe for use with patients. A major part of keeping care up to date is reviewing or evaluating literature on a subject. Evaluating research sounds rather daunting for the inexperienced but it can be broken down into a number of simple steps.

First, all research needs to be reliable (truthful) and valid (transferable), but not all research is necessarily relevant or applicable (Lindsay, 2007). Evidence sought needs to be linked directly to nurses' practice and to inform that practice, thereby making it relevant and applicable. Pearson (2000) is concerned that research results do not always relate to the reality of every-day practice. An example of this is a project where the use of ordinary tap water for wound cleansing was advocated. However, the study was carried out in a developed country where water is purified – the use of water in some countries would not be appropriate.

Secondly, nurses need to be critical of what evidence they use to inform their practice to enable them to decide the value or worth of a piece of research, given the purposes for which it is to be used. Hamer and Collinson (2005, p. 11) list qualities they believe are required for nurses to be 'critical', which are:

- to be questioning;

- to see more than one side of an argument;

- to be objective rather than subjective;

- to weigh evidence;

- to judge others' statements as being based on reason, evidence or logic on the one hand or based on partial evidence, special pleading, emotion or self-interest on the other;

- to look at the meaning behind the facts;

- to identify issues arising from the facts;

- to recognise when further evidence is needed.

Thirdly, nurses need to know how to evaluate a research article. Walsh (1997) states the decision (and ultimate accountability) lies with individual nurses to decide if the evidence they use is relevant, so they need the skills to evaluate the evidence critically. Below are some hints for evaluating research articles. This is a comprehensive guide to this process, but you may not be able to address all the points – it depends on the focus of the research article.

The article

**The title** – is it informative, interesting and to the point? i.e., does it address the question that you want answered?

**The authors** – what do you know about the authors? Do they have a vested interest in the conclusions of the study?

**The abstract** – does it summarise the main points of the study adequately and accurately? Be careful, as sometimes abstracts promise more than what is written in the rest of the paper.

**Introduction** – is the problem or purpose of the study clearly stated?

**The questions** – are they stated clearly and concisely? Do they follow logically from the problems? Are they worth answering? Are they answerable?

**The literature** – is the background information adequate? Does the author appear to know her/his subject? Does he/she appraise related research and authoritative statements? Or has he/she strung together citations and quotes which support her/his proposal without consideration of antagonistic arguments? Are specific theories used in order to put the study and potentially the findings into context? Does this theory seem relevant?

**Relevance** – is the study placed in the context of current professional knowledge? What is the potential contribution of the study to practice?

**Aims** – are the aims stated clearly, concisely and precisely? Are they logically related to the original question(s)? How were they formulated; for example, does evidence from the literature support intuition, instinct and experience? If treatment is being investigated, are the aims related to efficacy and safety?

The method

**Design** – is the study descriptive or experimental? Is it described adequately? Does the chosen design seem appropriate to you? A hypothesis or set of hypotheses is necessary for an experimental design. Does it follow logically from the original problem and theories?

**Assumptions** – are any assumptions being made? Is their use explained? Are they justifiable and appropriate? Was a pilot study completed, i.e. was a questionnaire or special report pre-tested for validity and reliability? Were modifications made? What were they and why?

**Ethical considerations** – has the author considered the ethics of the method? Is the proposed method ethically acceptable? For example, will all service users receive the treatment/intervention they need rather than the treatment needed for the study? Will a control group be required to receive a bogus or dummy treatment of dubious efficacy?

**Participants** – how were people selected? Are individuals allocated to alternative treatment/intervention groups? Is this ethical? Is there an account of how each person was chosen? Were specific criteria used to include or exclude people in and from the study? Are they clearly stated? Is the reasoning behind them apparent and sensible?

**Samples** – was a specific size of sample chosen (for example, for statistical purposes)? Does it seem adequate to provide sustainable results? If the author aims to make general comments about a population on the basis of the findings, who forms this population? Is the sample representative of this population?

**Data collection** – is the method described adequately? Could you replicate it from the description? Are the reasons for the choice of method stated? If special report forms, assessment forms, questionnaires or interview schedules have been used, are copies provided with the paper or is an address given for copies?

**Analysis** – is the method of analysis understandable? Have statistical tests been used? Are reasons for choice given which explain their appropriateness? Do you understand and accept the explanation?

**Results** – are results intelligible enough for you to interpret them and draw your own conclusions? Are they relevant to the stated problem? Does your background knowledge and common sense indicate that they are realistic and feasible? Are 'raw' data given, or only proportions, percentages, etc., after manipulation? Are histograms, pie charts and other graphic representations explained? Are the tables helpful? If results are based on responses to a questionnaire or interview schedule, what is the response rate? Are statistical results included? Are they meaningful? Is the statistical probability of results by chance included? Is it appropriate?

**Discussion** – are the results interpreted in relation to the original questions? Are the original questions answered? Have the aims been fulfilled? Does the author discuss any weaknesses in the methodology and factors which may have affected validity or reliability? For example, should sample selection be discussed? If criteria of inclusion and exclusion need clarification, is the explanation acceptable? Should the advantages and disadvantages of the method of data collection be discussed? Are they? Have you noticed anything that was omitted? Has the author referred to it or ignored it? Have the findings been related to the existing body of knowledge and relevant theory? Are the clinical implications discussed? Was the project funded? By whom? Might the results be biased because of the interests of the financing body?

**Conclusions** – how do they compare or contrast with the conclusions you drew from your interpretation of the results? Do they relate logically to the results?

**Recommendations** – are the recommendations self-evident from the reported results? Could you attempt to implement them, and should you? Is this study an end in itself, or does it suggest further research?

**References** – is the length of the list more impressive than its quality? Are any references conspicuous by their absence?

---

### ACTIVITY 7.2

- Go to the Research Mindedness website www.resmind.swap.ac.uk and click on the section 'are you research minded?', and undertake the self-evaluation questionnaire.

- Now find a research article in any nursing journal and review it, taking into account the above hints.

---

## Clinical effectiveness – does it work?

The term 'evidence-based practice' is often linked with clinical effectiveness. Williamson *et al.* (2008) believe clinical effectiveness is concerned with using treatments or care that have been shown to work, and it is important that what nurses do is effective because 'the NHS is a publicly funded service and it would be financially wasteful, pointless and immoral …to be using particular clinical interventions if they were not known to be effective' (Williamson *et al.*, 2008, p. 82).

The link between evidence-based practice and clinical effectiveness can be seen in the RCN's (1996b, p. 1) definition of clinical effectiveness: 'applying the best available knowledge, derived from research, clinical expertise and patient preferences, to achieve optimum processes and outcomes of care for patients' – a definition not dissimilar to the definition of evidence-based practice.

McClarey and Duff (1997) believe clinical effectiveness has three distinct parts – again not very different from evidence-based practice:

- **Obtaining evidence** – from research, either published in journals or available on databases; from national level studies based on research, for example, clinical guidelines, systematic reviews or national standards;

- **Implementing the evidence** – by changing practice to include the research evidence and, where possible, locally adapting national standards or guidelines;

- **Evaluating the impact of the changed practice** – and readjusting practice as necessary, usually through clinical audit and patient feedback.

Clinical effectiveness is also linked to clinical governance (see *Chapter 6*). Solomon (2003) states that clinical governance initiatives introduced by the government (Department of Health, 1998) aim to ensure that care provided is of high quality and has effective outcomes. These outcomes are achieved by employing the principles of evidence-based practice. Colyer and Kamath (1999, cited in Palfreyman *et al.*, 2003) add the economic benefits of evidence-based practice to their definition as they believe the overall purpose of evidence-based practice is to provide effective health care within the limited resources available. The Department of Health endorses this by saying demonstrating clinical and cost effectiveness is a key goal for the NHS (Department of Health, 1995; Department of Health, 1997) and one means of achieving this is evidence-based practice.

## Factors affecting the implementation of evidence-based practice

As indicated throughout this chapter, the use of evidence-based practice is critical to nurses, whether they be students or registered. However, Dougherty and Lister (2011) point out that, on the whole, delivering evidence-based care can be demanding and needs determination and time. Reasons for nurses not engaging in this practice have been cited by many authors, perhaps best summarised by Ciliska *et al.* (2001, p. 520) who say: 'barriers (to evidence-based practice) occur when time, access to journal articles, search skills, critical appraisal skills, and understanding of the language used in research are lacking'.

Other authors have also highlighted difficulties in engaging nurses in research and evidence-based practice (Gerrish and Lacey, 2006; Palfreyman *et al.*, 2003; Craig and Smyth, 2007). Some explanations for this are:

- The nature of evidence:

  - lack of clinically relevant research in nursing;

  - what do you do if there is no evidence?;

- tension between evidence and practice – where research unequivocally says that a particular practice, treatment or intervention works, and it doesn't;
- research is applied in a set of experimental conditions and cannot be reproduced in real life settings.

- How evidence is communicated:
  - often published in academic journals rather than professional journals which clinical nurses are more likely to read;
  - limited places at conferences where up-to-date information is presented;
  - language of research is sometimes a barrier;
  - researchers fail to draw out the implications of their research for practice.

- Knowledge and skills of individual nurses:
  - nurses do not have the knowledge and skills to access and appraise research information;
  - changing practice is exhausting – how often are nurses asked to do this?
  - changing practice involves accepting that you may have ceased to be right, and that you may not have been right for some time.

- Organisational barriers:
  - time, heavy clinical workloads;
  - lack of authority and support to implement findings;
  - implementing research in one area of practice may disrupt other area.

Finally, Lindsay (2007) reminds nurses that evidence is not only used to *change* practice, but it can also be used to support existing practice. Walsh (1997) believes research needs to be done by some, facilitated by others, and *implemented* by all.

### ACTIVITY 7.3

Choose a nursing duty and explore the literature about it. Then compare your findings with the practice you observe in your clinical area. Do they differ, and if so, what would you do about it?

> **FURTHER READING**
>
> This chapter does not attempt to discuss research methodologies, nor how to seek out literature – there are many textbooks that can help you with that. One such is Bruce Lindsay's *Understanding Research and Evidence-Based Practice*.

## Chapter summary

- All care given should be based on evidence-based practice.

- The care must be appropriate for the individual patient.

- Evidence-based practice is often linked with clinical effectiveness and clinical governance.

## References

Aveyard, H. & Sharp, P. (2009) *A Beginner's Guide to Evidence Based Practice in Health and Social Care*. Berkshire: Open University Press.

Bury, T. & Mead, J. (1998) *Evidence Based Health Care: A Practical Guide for Therapists*. Oxford: Butterworth-Heinemann.

Ciliska, D., Pinelli, J., DiCenso, A. & Cullum, N. (2001) Resources to enhance evidence-based nursing practice. *AACN Clinical Issues: Advanced Practice in Acute and Critical Care*, **12(4):** 520–528.

Colyer, H. & Kamath, P. (1999) Evidenced-based practice. A philosophical and political analysis: some matters for consideration by professional practitioners. *Journal of Advanced Nursing*, **29(1):** 188–193, cited in Palfreyman, S., Tod, S. & Doyle, J. (2003) An integrated approach to evidence-based practice. *The Foundation of Nursing Studies Dissemination Series*, **1(9):** 1–4.

Craig, J. & Smyth, R. (2007) *The Evidence-based Practice Manual for Nurses*. Edinburgh: Churchill Livingstone.

Dawes, M., Davies, P., Gray, A., Mant, J., Seers, K. & Snowball, R. (2005) *Evidence-based Practice: A Primer for Healthcare Professionals* (2nd edition). Edinburgh: Elsevier Churchill Livingstone.

Department of Health (1995) *Research and Development: Towards an Evidence-based Health Service*. London: HMSO.

Department of Health (1997) *The New NHS: Modern and Dependable*. London: HMSO.

Department of Health (1998) *A First Class Service: Quality in the New NHS*. London: HMSO.

Department of Health (2006) *Modernising Nursing Careers*. London: Department of Health.

Dougherty, L. & Lister, S. (2011) *The Royal Marsden Hospital Manual of Clinical Nursing Procedures* (8th edition). Chichester: Wiley-Blackwell.

Gerrish, K. & Lacey, A. (2006) *The Research Process in Nursing*. Oxford: Blackwell.

Hamer, S. & Collinson, G. (2005) *Achieving Evidence-Based Practice* (2nd edition). Edinburgh: Bailliere Tindall.

Higgs, J., Jones, M., Loftus, S. & Christensen, N. (2008) *Clinical Reasoning in the Health Professions* (3rd edition). Oxford: Butterworth-Heinemann.

Ingersoll, G. (2000) Evidence-based nursing: what it is and what it isn't. *Nursing Outlook*, **48(4):** 151–152.

Lindsay, B. (2007) *Understanding Research and Evidence-Based Practice*. Exeter: Reflect Press.

McClarey, M. & Duff, L. (1997) Clinical effectiveness and evidence-based practice. *Nursing Standard*, **11(52):** 31–35.

NHS Scotland (2005) *NHS Quality Improvement Scotland*. Available at www.clinicalgovernance.scot.nhs.uk/section5/qualityimprovement.asp (accessed 20 November 2012)

Nursing and Midwifery Council (2008) *The Code: Standards of Conduct, Performance and Ethics for Nurses and Midwives*. London: NMC.

Nursing and Midwifery Council (2010) *Standards for Pre-registration Nursing Education*. London: NMC.

Offredy, M. (2006) *Evidence-based Practice*, cited in Peate, I. (2006) *Becoming a Nurse in the 21st Century*. Chichester: John Wiley.

Palfreyman, S., Tod, S. & Doyle, J. (2003) An integrated approach to evidence-based practice. *The Foundation of Nursing Studies Dissemination Series*, **1(9):** 1–4.

Parahoo, K. (2006) *Nursing Research Principles, Process and Issues*. Basingstoke: Palgrave Macmillan.

Pearson, M. (2000) Making a difference through research: how nurses can turn the vision into reality (editorial). *Nursing Times Research*, **5(2):** 85–86.

Royal College of Nursing (1996a) *The Royal College of Nursing Clinical Effectiveness Initiative – A Strategic Framework*. London: RCN, cited in McClarey, M. & Duff, L. (1997) Clinical effectiveness and evidence-based practice. *Nursing Standard*, **11(52):** 31–35.

Royal College of Nursing (1996b) *Clinical Effectiveness*. London: RCN.

Rycroft-Malone, J., Seers, K., Titchen, A., Harvey, G., Kitson, A. & McCormack, B. (2004) What counts as evidence in evidence-based practice? *Journal of Advanced Nursing*, **47:** 81–90.

Sackett, D., Rosenberg, W., Gray, J., Haynes, R. & Richardson, W. (1996) Evidence-based medicine: what it is and what it isn't. *British Medical Journal*, **312:** 71–72.

Sackett, D., Richardson, S., Rosenberg, W. & Haynes, R. (2000) *Evidence-Based Medicine. How to Teach and Practice* (2nd edition). London: Churchill Livingstone.

Solomon, J. (2003) *Eating and Drinking*, cited in Holland, K., Jenkins, J., Solomon, J. & Whittam, S. (eds) *Roper, Logan and Tierney Model in Practice*. Edinburgh: Churchill Livingstone.

Walsh, M. (1997) How nurses perceive barriers to research implementation. *Nursing Standard*, **8(11):** 25–29.

Williamson, G., Jenkinson, T. & Proctor-Childs, T. (2008) *Nursing in Contemporary Healthcare Practice*. Exeter: Learning Matters.

www.resmind.swap.ac.uk (accessed 20 November 2012)

www.library.nhs.uk/Default.aspx (accessed 20 November 2012)

ebn.bmj.com (accessed 20 November 2012)

clinicalevidence.bmj.com/ceweb/index.jsp (accessed 20 November 2012)

www.thecochranelibrary.com (accessed 20 November 2012)

www.nice.org.uk (accessed 20 November 2012)

www.liv.ac.uk/mcpcil/liverpool-care-pathway (accessed 20 December 2012)

# 08

# INTERPROFESSIONAL PRACTICE
# AND CHANGING ROLES IN NURSING

The aim of this chapter is to provide a brief overview of interprofessional practice and changes in nurses' roles that have evolved since the late 1990s.

**Learning Outcomes**

On completion of this chapter you should be able to:

- understand the concept and context of interprofessional practice
- appraise the role and function of relevant health and social care professionals
- appreciate why there has been a need for nurses' roles to change
- understand the main changes that have occurred to nurses' roles in the past decade.

## Interprofessional practice

The push towards interprofessional collaboration in the field of health care is relatively new and although there is a professional consensus that it is a positive ideal, it appears to be largely politically driven. As you would expect, since 1948 the provision of health care in the United Kingdom (UK) has undergone a variety of changes in terms of organisational restructuring, managerial and economic change. Many of these changes have unfortunately resulted in the fragmentation of health and social care services. This includes those services that are managed at local level through different governmental channels, each having different funding arrangements and dissimilar involvement with independent and voluntary sector care. In addition to this, professional cultures and forms of accountability within each of the groups have tended to differ significantly.

A perceived solution to this problem by the government has been the attempt, through legislation and initiatives, to develop services at local level that are integrated and require members of different professions and agencies to work together to develop and improve the provision and delivery of health care services. This principle has been central to health and social care provision and delivery policy since the early 1990s and has survived changes of government.

The issues raised in this chapter will have relevance for wherever you work in the UK.

## Definitions

There are a number of terms associated with or used in the context of inter-professional practice. The following are those you are most likely to come into contact with.

- **Uni-disciplinary** – professional groups work independently of one another.

- **Multiprofessional/multidisciplinary** – as with uni-disciplinary practice, professional groups tend to function independently of one another, but some discussion and negotiation does on occasion occur in order to solve problems outside the scope of the traditional and established professional disciplines.

- **Intraprofessional/intradisciplinary** – a professional group that is further divided into smaller sections, each with its own specific area of specialism such as, for example, nursing – adult, paediatric, mental health, health visiting, district nursing. Intersecting lines of communication and collaboration exist between these professional specialisms.

- **Interprofessional/interdisciplinary** – intersecting lines of communication and collaboration between different professions and agencies (for example, health and social care, nursing and allied health professionals); the groups are more integrated and all modify their efforts to take account of other team members' contributions (Leathard, 2003; Day, 2007; College of Nurses Ontario, 2008).

- **Collaboration** – can simply mean 'work jointly on an activity or project' (Pearsall, 2001).

> **ACTIVITY 8.1**
>
> Consider each of the definitions above and try to relate it to any previous experi-
> ence you may have had in a care/work environment.

## Benefits of interprofessional practice

A review of the literature (Leathard, 2003; Barrett *et al.*, 2005; Hammick
*et al.*, 2009) suggests there is a general consensus, not only in the political
arena but also among health and social care professionals, that interprofessional practice can be a positive thing and should provide many benefits to
both the practitioners involved and the clients/patients they care for. The
identified benefits of such practice include that it:

- allows for streamlining of services (government driven);

- provides for a more effective use of staff;

- offers increased overall quality of service provision;

- provides better use of limited resources.

For the practitioners involved, interprofessional practice also:

- provides a more satisfying work environment;

- can encourage development of mutual respect, mutual co-operation and
  empathy between professionals;

- should improve communication between different professionals;

- allows all members of the team to understand each others' roles and
  recognise areas of overlap within the traditional disciplines;

- can encourage a greater understanding of the difference between
  accountability and responsibility of different team members and what is
  expected of them.

For service users, benefits include:

- continuity of care;

- consistency of care;

- decrease of ambiguity in the information being given to the patient;

- appropriate referral because of the greater understanding of other professionals' roles;

- care being based on a holistic perspective with the best-placed professionals to meet this agenda.

(Miller *et al.*, 2001)

According to Barrett *et al.* (2005), if such benefits of interprofessional practice are to be maximised, not only will it require complex interactions between practitioners, but certain other factors and processes will also need to be in place. These include:

- knowledge of professional roles;

- willing participation;

- open and honest communication;

- trust and mutual respect;

- shared power;

- confidence;

- support and commitment at a senior level.

## Knowledge of professional roles

In order for effective interprofessional practice to take place, it is considered essential that each team member has an understanding of the role and professional boundaries of other practitioners they may be working with.

### ACTIVITY 8.2

You may already be participating in shared learning with other professional groups – in particular, physiotherapy, occupational therapy and radiography students. Take some time to talk to them about their specific role and function within the care environment.

Other care professionals that you will be involved with during your training include the following.

## District nurse (family health nurse)

A district nurse must be qualified and registered in adult nursing and have undertaken a specialist practitioner programme (minimum first-degree level). These programmes are normally no less than one academic year (32 weeks) full-time or part-time equivalent (although it may be completed in a shorter period of time where credit is given for prior learning). Community staff nurses can be funded onto the specialist programme via their individual employer.

District nurses are an integral part of the primary health care team. They provide nursing care to patients during periods of illness / incapacity in non-hospital settings. This is usually in the patient's own home but can also be in residential care homes, health centres or general practitioner surgeries. Patients may be of any age and include those who are housebound, elderly, terminally ill, disabled and those recently discharged from hospital. Their work is diverse but their main activities include:

- accepting referrals from other professionals and agencies such as, for example, hospitals and general practitioners;

- assessing, planning and managing the care of patients;

- establishing links with patients' families and carers and, where appropriate, working with them to develop their skills in caring for the patient;

- working both intra- and interprofessionally with a range of other professionals and agencies within the National Health Service (NHS), social care, independent and voluntary sector;

- playing a fundamental role in promoting healthy lifestyles and health education / teaching;

- prescribing from an identified list.

(www.nhscareers.nhs.uk; www.prospects.ac.uk)

## Health visitor

A health visitor must be a qualified and registered nurse (in adult, child, mental health or learning disabilities) or midwife, and have undertaken an approved specialist community public health nursing (health visiting) programme (SCPHN/HV). The programmes normally comprise 45 weeks' study to be completed within a 156-week period (part-time study should be completed within 208 weeks). Accreditation of prior learning can be applied to a maximum of one-third of a SCPHN/HV programme. Course funding is usually through the individual's employer, although a few people may fund themselves.

Health visitors are usually part of the primary health care team and their role involves working in clinics and doctors' surgeries, as well as visiting people in their own homes. Health visitors undertake a range of work including:

• leading and delivering child and family health services (pregnancy through to five years);

• providing ongoing additional services for vulnerable children and families;

• contributing to multidisciplinary services in safeguarding and protecting children;

• focusing on the prevention and early detection of ill health and the promotion of healthy lifestyles;

• participating in the design, implementation and evaluation of public health programmes.

(www.nhscareers.nhs.uk; nursingcareers.nhsemployers.org; www.prospects.ac.uk)

## Social worker

A qualified social worker will have undertaken a professional qualification at degree or postgraduate level and be registered with a Care Council (as appropriate for England, Scotland, Wales or Northern Ireland). Currently, funding for the student to undertake the education / training may come from employer sponsorship, a bursary or the individual.

Social workers practise in a variety of settings including service users' homes, schools, hospitals and other public-sector and voluntary organisations. They work with all age groups and support individuals, families and groups in the community within a framework of relevant legislation and procedures, as well as working closely with other organisations including those providing health care. They offer support, advice, counselling and protection to all age groups, although they may choose to specialise in one specific area. In England, social workers tend to specialise in either children or adult services.

Working with children and families

This area can include:

- working to protect children believed to be at risk;

- assisting parents who are experiencing difficulties with bringing up their child / children;

- managing the fostering or adoption process for children who cannot be cared for by their own families;

- helping to keep families together (providing advice and support);

- working with children in care homes;

- working with young offenders in the community.

Working with adults

This area can involve:

- evaluating the needs of vulnerable older people in the community and developing care plans that enable the client to remain living safely and independently at home;

- supporting adults who have offended, through supervision or helping with resettlement;

- working with specific groups such as people with HIV or AIDS, adults with mental illness, physical disabilities or learning difficulties;

- working to protect vulnerable adults.

In Northern Ireland, Wales, and Scotland, social workers can choose to specialise in a wider range of front line services.

(www.hpc-uk.org; www.basw.co.uk; www.nhscareers.nhs.uk)

# Willing participation

High levels of motivation and willingness of the participants are pivotal to the effectiveness of any interprofessional collaboration. Maintaining such motivation and willingness, even if unsatisfactory experiences of interprofessional practice are encountered, is very important (Molyneux, 2001; Pollard, 2009).

## Confidence

Writers such as Leathard (2003) suggest that the most basic requirement for interprofessional collaboration must be the individual's own professional competence. They argue that until the practitioner feels confident that they are experts in their own field, and are regarded as such by their peers, they are unlikely to feel sufficiently secure to engage fully in sharing practice with others outside their own professional arena. Personal levels of confidence within the practice area will increase as you progress through your student nurse programme and after you qualify.

## Open and honest communication

Open and honest communication is linked very closely to internal feelings associated with an individual's level of confidence. It also involves the need for the participants to set aside any assumptions and judgements they may have about other professions involved in the collaborative practice (Interprofessional Education Collaborative Panel, 2011).

## Trust and mutual respect

Trust can be viewed as a vital characteristic of collaboration, and another component that develops over time through repeated positive interprofessional experiences, both in the classroom and in practice. Mutual respect, according to Barrett *et al.* (2005), develops when, again, all participants feel valued through explicit acknowledgement of each profession's unique contribution to the overall process.

## Shared power

Shared power, in this context, is seen as being based on non-hierarchical relationships. Historically, power tended to be located within the medical profession; however, with ever-increasing advanced nursing roles, this does appear to be changing.

## Support and commitment at a senior level

According to Fieldgrass (1992, cited in Barrett *et al.*, 2005), commitment to interprofessional working must also occur at a senior level as collaborative practice can be expensive in terms of time and resources. If such practice is imposed from senior level then support for the professionals involved in its development must also come from that level. This, according to Barrett *et al.*

(2005), needs to involve such strategies as encouraging reflection through clinical supervision, education and training, team development and establishing the guidelines relating to the parameters within which individual professions work.

## Postscript and a note of caution

Despite the recognised benefits there are still some difficulties with, and barriers to effective and widespread interprofessional practice, particularly within health and social care. These include:

- **organisational issues** – between health and social services, such as, for example, disparity of boundaries (both geographical and professional) and centres of control;

- **operational matters** – different budgetary and planning sequences and procedures;

- **monetary factors** – including different funding structures and sources of financial resources;

- **status and validity** – social care is directed through democratically elected and appointed agencies, i.e. local authorities, whereas health care is directed by policy from central government through the NHS;

- **professional issues** are numerous and include:

  - problems associated with differing ideologies, values and language;

  - conflicting views about users;

  - separate training backgrounds;

  - differing organisational boundaries and professional loyalties;

  - inequalities in status and pay;

  - lack of clarity about roles and historical prejudices;

  - professional defence of professions and an unwillingness to dilute them in any way (professional protectionism);

  - differences between specialisms, expertise and skills – this can include medical practitioners (and can occur intraprofessionally as well as interprofessionally).

(Leathard, 2003; Day, 2007; www.med.mun.ca)

However, ongoing government policy, legislation and directives and the inclusion of interprofessional education and training for health and social care professionals all seek to lessen the impact of the above factors.

> **FURTHER READING**
>
> Discussion of a range of issues associated with interprofessional practice can be found both online and through journals such as the *Journal of Interprofessional Care*, which promotes collaboration in education, practice and research for health and social care, and the *Journal of Research in Interprofessional Practice and Education*, which disseminates theoretical perspectives, methodologies and evidence-based knowledge to inform interprofessional practice.

# Changing roles in nursing

## Why the need for change?

The International Council of Nurses (2010) offers a definition of nursing that encompasses the vast arena of care that nurses deliver. While it is accepted that not all nurses are involved in all the aspects of nursing described at any one time, nurses still need to be flexible, adaptable and innovative in order to respond to the changing needs and perceptions of their patients. In addition, a market-driven health service and ever-changing reforms require their role to be continuously evolving and changing.

> **THE ICN DEFINITION OF NURSING**
>
> Nursing encompasses autonomous and collaborative care of individuals of all ages, families, groups and communities, sick or well and in all settings. Nursing includes the promotion of health, prevention of illness, and the care of ill, disabled and dying people. Advocacy, promotion of a safe environment, research, participation in shaping health policy and in patient and health systems management, and education are also key nursing roles (ICN, 2010).

## The NHS Plan

Probably the most profound impact on a nurse's work life in recent years has been the introduction of *The NHS Plan* (Department of Health, 2000). This has since been superseded by other government initiatives, but at the time, *The Plan* represented the biggest change to health care in England since the NHS was formed in 1948. Along with setting out reform of the NHS, it included a section on the roles nurses should undertake and 'encouraged nurses and other staff to extend their roles'.

Many of the changes in the health service today, which include the role of the nurse, have been driven by patients. Patient perceptions and expectations of their health care have risen as information on medical and nursing roles have been made more accessible and transparent. However, the changing roles of other health care professionals (particularly changes resulting from the European Working Time Directive) have also had an impact on the nurse's role, and in some instances have led to the creation of new roles altogether for nurses.

## Changing policy, changing practice (NMC, 2005)

The NMC has summarised the changes in the registered nurse's role over the past decades (*see below*). Although currently a student, you need to have an awareness of changes in the role you will assume once registered, and of your future professional body's viewpoint on this:

> The practice of nurses, midwives and health visitors is constantly evolving and changing. Nurses, midwives and health visitors have continually adjusted the scope of their practice to meet changing health needs. Changes in health policy, such as the shift towards a primary care led NHS, an increasing emphasis on public health and community based services, together with technological advances and developments in scientific knowledge have required all the health care professions to develop in new ways. These changes have increased the skills and decision-making required of all nurses, midwives and health visitors. What was once unthinkable – nurses carrying out endoscopies, acting as specialists in diverse areas of care such as diabetes and behavioural therapy, working as first assistant to surgeons, and running their own clinics in acute and primary care; midwives developing and leading total programmes of care for pregnant women with severe social and/or emotional

difficulties, directing the development of clinical guidelines, and specialising in supporting women and their partners following early pregnancy loss; health visitors co-ordinating community development work, specialising in child protection, and leading multi-agency work on service development for older people – is now becoming commonplace. *The scope of professional practice* encouraged nurses, midwives and health visitors to take on new roles and activities to adapt to meet changing health care needs. There are few tasks which nurses, midwives and health visitors cannot undertake legally and many former 'extended role' activities, e.g. intravenous drug administration, cannulation, venepuncture and ECGs now form the expected skill base of all registered practitioners.

The clinical nurse specialist role in areas such as infection control, tissue viability, stoma care, continence and so on has existed informally since the 1970s. Clinical nurse specialists were seen as experts in a particular area of care or with a particular client group, with post-qualification education and a research base firmly grounded in nursing. The title was not regulated and post-holders usually achieved such jobs through extensive experience and appropriate post-registration courses. Clinical nurse specialists were usually managed within the nursing service. Nurse practitioners developed first in primary care in the late 1980s and offered an alternative service to that provided by general practitioners or filled gaps in service provision such as providing primary care to homeless people. Nurse practitioners diagnose, refer, prescribe and provide complete episodes of care for clients with undifferentiated health problems. In the 1990s, posts emerged in secondary care with the titles of nurse practitioner, advanced practitioner and advanced nurse practitioner. Such posts frequently involve nurses giving care or performing tasks previously done by doctors. For example, in some trusts advanced neo-natal practitioners are replacing junior doctors on the senior house officer rota in special care baby units; surgical nurse practitioners run pre-admission clinics, clerk patients and organise theatre lists, other nurse practitioners work across the primary / secondary care interface and prescribe within protocols for conditions such as hypertension, asthma and so on.

Latterly, consultant nurse, midwife and health visitor posts have been introduced in the NHS. Consultant nurses, midwives and health visitors are expected to be competent to initiate and lead significant practice, education and service development.

Four key areas of responsibility have been defined – expert practice; professional leadership and consultancy; education and development; and practice and service development linked to research and evaluation.

Consultant nurses, midwives and health visitors are to have been educated to masters or doctorate level, be registered as a nurse, midwife or health visitor, and hold additional professional qualifications. The development of such posts has been described as a national priority and it has been suggested that these posts should be used to tackle particular service problems and lead service development in government determined priority areas.

In the past, registration was seen as a licence to practise for life. In today's world however the importance of all practitioners ensuring that their skills and expertise remain relevant to the needs of their patients and clients and constantly learning and updating their knowledge and skills is increasingly recognised.

In light of the increasing speed and nature of change in the professional practice of many nurses, midwives and health visitors outlined above, the NMC recognised and responded to the need to consider how its regulatory frameworks protected the public.

(NMC, 2005)

## ACTIVITY 8.3

Having read the NMC statement above, list any specialist roles you have seen undertaken by nurses in your placement areas.

## New nursing roles

One of the reasons nurses' roles are changing is that the organisations within health care have also had to change the way they work, in order to accommodate new technologies, new legislation (both UK and European) and new government initiatives. Some of these new roles nurses are now undertaking are considered below. This is not an exhaustive list, but highlights the concept of nurses working beyond their initial registration:

### Nurse consultants

Nurse consultant posts were first established in 1999. They are central to the process of health service modernisation, helping to provide patients with services that are fast and convenient. Nurse consultants are very experienced registered nurses, who will specialise in a particular field of health care. Each consultant role will be very different, depending on the needs of the employer, but nurses working at this level are amongst the highest paid of their professions.

All nurse consultants spend a minimum of 50 per cent of their time working directly with patients, ensuring that people using the NHS continue to benefit from the very best nursing skills. In addition, they are responsible for developing personal practice, being involved in research and evaluation and contributing to education, training and development (www.nhscareers.nhs.uk).

### Advanced nurse practitioner

The National Health Service Executive's strategic document *Making a Difference – Strengthening the Nursing, Midwifery and Health Visiting Contribution to Health and Health Care* (Department of Health, 1999a) outlined a new career framework for nurses. This framework includes the development of advanced nursing posts that are intended to extend the career opportunities for expert nurses who wish to remain in clinically focused roles.

The advanced nurse practitioner is one of these posts, and can be found in both primary and secondary care settings. The NMC (2006) defines the role thus:

> Advanced Nurse Practitioners are highly experienced and educated members of the care team who are able to diagnose and treat (your) healthcare needs or refer (you) to an appropriate specialist if needed.

The Royal College of Nursing (2010) further defines an advanced nurse practitioner as:

> A registered nurse who has undertaken a specific course of study of at least first degree (honours) level and who:
>
> - makes professional autonomous decisions, for which he or she is accountable;

- receives patients with undifferentiated and undiagnosed problems and makes an assessment of their health care needs, based on highly developed nursing knowledge and skills, including skills not usually exercised by nurses, such as physical examination;

- screens patients for disease risk factors and early signs of illness;

- makes a differential diagnosis using decision-making and problem-solving skills;

- develops with the patient an ongoing nursing care plan for health, with an emphasis on preventative measures;

- orders necessary investigations, and provides treatment and care both individually, as part of a team, and through referral to other agencies;

- has a supportive role in helping people to manage and live with illness;

- provides counselling and health education;

- has the authority to admit or discharge patients from their caseload, and refer patients to other health care providers as appropriate;

- works collaboratively with other health care professionals and disciplines;

- provides a leadership and consultancy function as required.

For further information about the role of advanced nurse practitioners visit www.rcn.org.uk and type 'advanced nurse practitioners' into the search engine.

### Nurse prescriber

Since 1994 some nurses have been able to prescribe medicines for certain groups of patients. In 1999 the *Review of Prescribing, Supply and Administration of Medicines* (Department of Health, 1999b) put forward key principles for the extension of prescribing rights. These principles included the need for appropriate training, regulation and updating, and the need for prescribing to take place within a framework of accountability and competency.

In 2008 the NMC further clarified who could prescribe what, and what qualifications were required:

Qualified nurse prescribers (NMC, 2008, Standard 1)

The Medicinal Products: Prescription by Nurses Act (1992) and subsequent amendments allow nurses who have recorded their qualification on the NMC register to become nurse prescribers. There are two levels of prescribers:

**Community practitioner nurse prescribers**: These are registrants who have successfully undertaken a programme of preparation to prescribe from the nurse prescribers' formulary for community practitioners. They can prescribe the majority of dressings and appliances, and a limited range of prescription-only medicines. The Nurse Prescribers' Formulary for Community Practitioners can be found on the British National Formulary website, www.bnf.org (you will need to register for this website, but it is free).

**Independent and supplementary nurse and midwife prescribers**: These are nurses and midwives who are trained to make a diagnosis and prescribe the appropriate treatment (independent prescribing). They may also, in cases where a doctor has made an initial diagnosis, go on to prescribe or review the medication, and change the drug, dosage, timing or frequency, or route of administration of any medication as appropriate, as part of a clinical management plan (supplementary prescribing).

Nurse or midwife independent prescribers can prescribe all prescription-only medicines including some controlled drugs, and all medication that can be supplied by a pharmacist or bought over the counter. However, they must only prescribe drugs that are within their area of expertise and level of competence, and should only prescribe for children if they have the expertise and competence to do so. Additionally they must comply with current prescribing legislation and are accountable for their practice.

For Department of Health guidance visit www.dh.gov.uk and search for 'nurse independent prescribing'.

### Modern Matrons

Modern Matrons (from: *Modern Matrons – Improving the Patient Experience*, Department of Health, 2003) were introduced in the mid-2000s to provide strong leadership on wards and be highly visible and accessible to patients. They lead by example in driving up standards of clinical care and empower nurses to take on a greater range of clinical tasks to help improve patient care. Crucially, they also have the power to get the basics right for patients – clean wards, good food, quality care.

The new matron role positions nursing at the very heart of the NHS modernisation process. It is part of a profound cultural change which puts the patient first. In such a system, effective front-line leaders are vitally important in achieving delivery.

Their ten key responsibilities are:

- leading by example;

- making sure patients get quality care;

- ensuring staffing is appropriate to patient needs;

- empowering nurses to take on a wider range of clinical tasks;

- improving hospital cleanliness;

- ensuring patients' nutritional needs are met;

- improving wards for patients;

- making sure patients are treated with respect;

- preventing hospital-acquired infection;

- resolving problems for patients and their relatives by building closer relationships.

### *Assistant Practitioner*

In addition to enhancing the role of registered nurses, a new grade of Assistant Practitioner was introduced in the mid-2000s. Assistant Practitioners work in a broad range of areas, primarily but not exclusively with patient contact. In clinical areas, they will usually be managed by a health care professional; for example a dietician, nurse, occupational therapist, midwife, physiotherapist, operating department practitioner or health care scientist. The exact role will vary, depending upon the area they work in.

The Assistant Practitioner role is at Level 4 of the Career Framework. Assistant Practitioners are required to have a level of knowledge and skill beyond that of the traditional health care assistant or support worker. They would be able to deliver elements of health and social care and undertake clinical work in domains that were previously only within the remit of registered professionals. They are accountable to themselves, their employer and, more importantly, the people they serve (www.skillsforhealth.org.uk).

General responsibilities of an Assistant Practitioner may include:

- planning, delivering and evaluating delegated care within clear protocols;
- delivering delegated health promotion initiatives and advice;
- assisting in identifying health needs of patients;
- maintaining clear and accurate patient records;
- a range of physiological measurements;
- venepuncture and cannulation;
- routine catheterisation.

## Chapter summary

- There is a general consensus both in the political arena and among care professionals that interprofessional practice is a positive action for both practitioners and service users.

- High levels of motivation and willingness of the participants are pivotal to the effectiveness of any interprofessional collaboration.

- Despite the recognised benefits, there are some difficulties with, and barriers to effective and widespread interprofessional practice, particularly with health and social care.

- There are a number of advanced practice roles which registered nurses can train for after registration.

## References

Barrett, G., Sellman, D. & Thomas, J. (2005) *Multi-disciplinary Working in Health Care and Social Care – Professional Perspectives.* Basingstoke: Palgrave Macmillan.

College of Nurses Ontario (2008) *Interprofessional Collaboration among Health Colleges and Professions.* Available from www.hprac.org/en/projects/resources/hprac-1433May28CollegeOfNurses.pdf (accessed 20 November 2012)

Day, J. (2007) *Interprofessional Working*. Hampshire: Cengage Learning.

Department of Health (1999a) *Making a Difference – Strengthening the Nursing, Midwifery and Health Visiting Contribution to Health and Health Care*. London: Department of Health.

Department of Health (1999b) *Review of Prescribing, Supply and Administration of Medicines*. London: Department of Health.

Department of Health (2000) *The NHS Plan*. London: Department of Health.

Department of Health (2003) *Modern Matrons – Improving the Patient Experience*. London: Department of Health.

Hammick, M., Freeth, D., Copperman, J. & Goddsman, D. (2009) *Being Interprofessional*. Cambridge: Polity Press.

International Council of Nurses (2010) *Definition of Nursing*. Geneva: ICN.

Interprofessional Education Collaborative Panel (2011) *Core Competencies for Interprofessional Collaborative Practice: Report of Expert Panel*. Washington, DC: Interprofessional Education Collaborative. Available from www.aacn.nche.edu/education-resources/ipecreport.pdf (accessed 20 November 2012)

Leathard, A. (2003) *Interprofessional Collaboration: From Policy to Practice in Health and Social Care*. Hove: Brunner-Routledge.

Miller, C., Freeman, M. & Ross, N. (2001) *Interprofessional Practice in Health and Social Care: Challenging the Shared Learning Agenda*. London: Arnold.

Molyneux, J. (2001) Multi-disciplinary teamworking: what makes teams work well? *Journal of Multi-disciplinary Care*, **15:** 29–35.

Nursing and Midwifery Council (2005) *Changing Policy, Changing Practice*. London: NMC.

Nursing and Midwifery Council (2006) *A Revision of the Definition of Advanced Nurse Practice so that it could be Accessible to Patients and the Public*. London: NMC.

Nursing and Midwifery Council (2008) *Standards for Medicines Management*. London: NMC.

Pearsall, J. (ed.) (2001) *The Concise Oxford Dictionary* (10th edition). Oxford: Oxford University Press.

Pollard, K. (2009) Student engagement in interprofessional working in practice placement settings. *Journal of Clinical Nursing,* **18(20):** 2856–2856.

Royal College of Nursing (2010) *Advanced Nurse Practitioners – an RCN Guide to the Advanced Nurse Practitioner Role, Competencies and Programme Accreditation* (revised). London: RCN.

www.basw.co.uk/social-work-careers (accessed 20 November 2012)

www.nhscareers.nhs.uk/details/Default.aspx?ID = 78 (accessed 20 November 2012)

www.nhscareers.nhs.uk/details/Default.aspx?Id = 519 (accessed 20 November 2012)

http://nursingcareers.nhsemployers.org/browse-segments/family-and-public-health/level-6-clinical/specialist-practitioner-health-visitor-public-health.aspx (accessed 14 January 2013)

www.nmc-uk.org (accessed 20 November 2012)

www.prospects.ac.uk/health_visitor_job_description.htm (accessed 20 November 2012)

http://ww2.prospects.ac.uk/p/types_of_job/district_nurse_job_description.jsp%20 (accessed 14 January 2013)

www.hpc-uk.org (accessed 14 January 2013)

www.med.mun.ca/getdoc/5662c96a-7a26-4fcf-b19c-ccb806a5df44/Common-barriers-to-interprofessional-healthcare-te.aspx (accessed 20 November 2012)

www.dh.gov.uk (accessed 20 November 2012)

www.icn.ch/definition.htm (accessed 20 November 2012)

www.nhscareers.nhs.uk (accessed 20 November 2012)

www.nmc-uk.org (accessed 20 November 2012)

www.skillsforhealth.org.uk (accessed 20 November 2012)

# 09
## REFLECTION AND PROFESSIONAL DEVELOPMENT

This chapter looks at reflection as a learning strategy and how it informs two specific aspects of professional development: clinical supervision and portfolios.

| **Learning Outcomes** | |
|---|---|
| On completion of this chapter you should be able to: | • understand the concept of reflection as a learning strategy; |
| | • describe the process of reflection and exercise the skills required to carry this out; |
| | • discuss the advantages of using reflection in practice; |
| | • appreciate how the reflective skills you develop as a student are carried on into registered nurse practice; |
| | • have an understanding of the need to maintain a portfolio; |
| | • appreciate the NMC's position on personal professional profiles; |
| | • consider how you might structure your own portfolio; |
| | • appreciate the concept and advantages of clinical supervision. |

## Reflection

Reflection is associated with learning from experience and is viewed as an important strategy for nurses, who should all embrace life-long learning. The term 'reflection' is often used synonymously with the terms 'reflective practice' and 'reflective learning', and the literature about reflection indicates that most agree it is an active, conscious process where an experience is explored in order to gain new understandings and to learn something new. Dewey stated this as long ago as 1938 when he simply said: 'we learn by doing and realising what we did' (Dewey, 1938, cited in Jasper, 2006). Moon (2004) agrees with this when stating that reflective learning is where the learner considers their practice honestly and critically and is often initiated when the individual practitioner encounters some problematic aspect of practice and attempts to make sense of it. However, Jasper (2006, p. 44) makes the distinction between reflection and reflective practice: 'using reflection alone in order to learn is not reflective practice... practice is about doing something. Therefore reflective practice means using the reflective process to inform practice in some way'.

Jasper (2006) also points out that reflection is a learning strategy that can be achieved either formally or informally and can be outside the formal learning environment. It can help bridge the theory–practice gap that students often find so challenging: as a student you develop skills for learning in an educational setting (analysing literature, writing essays, etc.) whereas in practice you learn from the clinical setting, by working with your mentor and other healthcare professionals, performing new skills, assessing patients' needs, planning their care, etc. Reflection can help integrate these learning processes by using the theory gained from the educational setting to inform everyday working practices.

There are many different models for reflection, with no one being better than any other – it is a matter of personal choice which is used, but the consensus from nursing literature is that reflection should be structured to enable learning to result from it. Price (2002) suggests that reflection is more comfortable and effective if a step-by-step approach is used, and most of the reflective models acknowledge this with a broad outline of the stages being:

- thinking back over a situation;

- possibly discussing the incident with other people;

- re-evaluating the experience to seek possible new understandings;

- checking out new knowledge;

- developing an action plan for the future.

(Whitehead and Mason, 2007)

Good reflective practice underpins good professional practice in that reflection enables practitioners to review their progress and identify areas which have been successfully developed, and those which are in need of further development. It enhances a commitment to 'life-long learning' and continuous professional development (Somerset Academy, 2005).

# Models of reflection

As mentioned above, there are many models of reflection to choose from. Outlined below are three of the most widely used:

## Gibbs' reflective cycle

Gibbs' (1998) reflective cycle (see *Figure 9.1*) is fairly straightforward and encourages a clear description of the situation, analysis of feelings, evaluation of the experience, analysis to make sense of the experience, conclusion where other options are considered, and reflection upon experience to examine what you would do if the situation arose again.

### Stage 1: Description of the event

Describe in detail the event you are reflecting on. Include, for example, where were you; who else was there; why were you there; what were you doing; what were other people doing; the context of the event; what happened; what was your part in this; what parts did the other people play; what was the result?

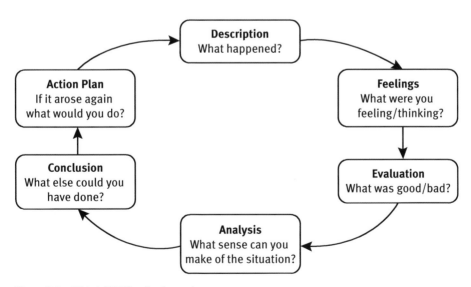

*Figure 9.1 – Gibbs' (1998) reflective cycle*

### Stage 2: Feelings

At this stage try to recall and explore the things that were going on inside your head, i.e. why does this event stick in your mind? Include, for example: how were you feeling when the event started; what were you thinking about at the time; how did it make you feel; how did other people make you feel; how did you feel about the outcome of the event; what do you think about it now?

### Stage 3: Evaluation

Try to evaluate or make a judgement about what has happened. Consider what was good about the experience and what didn't go so well or was bad about the experience.

### Stage 4: Analysis

Break the event down into its component parts so they can be explored separately. You may need to ask more detailed questions about the answers to the last stage. Include, for example: what went well; what did you do well; what did others do well; what went wrong or did not turn out how it should have done; in what way did you or others contribute to this?

### Stage 5: Conclusion

This differs from the evaluation stage in that you have now explored the issue from different angles and have a lot of information on which to base your judgement. It is here that you are likely to develop insight into your own and other people's behaviour in terms of how they contributed to the outcome of the event. Remember the purpose of reflection is to learn from an experience. Without detailed analysis and honest exploration that occurs during all the previous stages, it is unlikely that all aspects of the event will be taken into account and therefore valuable opportunities for learning can be missed. During this stage you should ask yourself what you could have done differently.

### Stage 6: Action plan

During this stage you should think yourself forward into encountering the event again and plan what you would do – would you act differently or would you be likely to do the same?

Here the cycle is tentatively completed and suggests that, should the event occur again, it will be the focus of another reflective cycle.

## Johns' (2006) model for structured reflection: Version 15

Johns' (2006, cited in Johns, 2010) model for structured reflection can be used as a guide for analysis of a critical incident or general reflection on experience, and is useful for more complex analyses. Johns believes that the reflector should work with a supervisor as he considers that through sharing reflections, greater understanding of those experiences can be achieved, rather than the reflector undertaking a lone exercise.

The stages of Johns' model of structured reflection are:

- bring the mind home
- focus on a description that seems significant in some way
- what particular issues seem significant to pay attention to?
- how were others feeling and what made them feel that way?
- how was I feeling and what made me feel that way?
- what was I trying to achieve and did I respond effectively?
- what were the consequences of my actions on the patient, others, myself?
- what factors influenced the way I was feeling, thinking and responding?
- what knowledge did inform or might have informed me?
- to what extent did I act for the best and in tune with my values?
- how does this situation connect with previous experience?
- how might I respond more effectively given this situation again?
- what would be the consequences of alternative actions for the patient, others and myself?
- what factors might constrain me acting in new ways?
- how do I now feel about this experience?
- am I more able to support myself and others better as a consequence?
- am I more able to realise desirable practice?

## Stephenson's reflective model (1993)

Another very useful framework was developed by a nursing student (Stephenson, 1993, cited in Palmer *et al.*, 1994) as a result of four years' experience of reflecting on her practice. This framework takes a critical approach, moving from personal reflection to consideration of ethical, political and social issues. Essentially Stephenson's framework involves considering:

- what was my role in this situation?

- did I feel comfortable or uncomfortable – why?

- what actions did I take?

- how did I and others act?

- was it appropriate?

- how could I have improved the situation for myself, the patient, my mentor?

- what can I achieve in the future?

- do I feel as if I have learnt anything new about myself?

- did I expect anything different to happen – what and why?

- has it changed my way of thinking in any way?

- what knowledge from theory and research can I apply to this situation?

- what broader issues, for example ethical, political or social, arise from this situation?

- what do I think about these broader issues?
  (Stephenson, 1993, cited in Palmer *et al.*, 1994, pp. 56–57)

## Using reflective frameworks

Regardless of which model for reflection is used, Price (2002) suggests that the challenge of using reflective frameworks is often in ensuring that you have considered the following:

- did you consider your own prejudices?

- did you avoid seeing only the familiar and/or one perspective?

- did you consider what others might have intended to signal through their behaviour?

- did you make use of and check out all the available information?

- did you actually learn something new?

- did you form an action plan of how to approach this differently in future?

## The benefits of practising reflectively

Jasper (2006, p. 53) lists the people and organisations she believes benefit from nurses practising reflectively. They are:

- the individual, in terms of providing individualised care, identifying their learning needs, and learning from experience;

- the patient, in terms of higher quality and standards of care, and care designed to meet their own unique needs;

- the employer, in terms of standards of care achieved, in having a continually developing workforce which recognises its own professional development;

- the profession, in terms of self-regulation of the practitioners, in developing the nursing knowledge base, in contributing to increasing the status of nursing and recognition of nurses' contribution to patient care.

### ACTIVITY 9.1

To see if Gibbs' reflective cycle can help you reflect on aspects of your practice, recall a recent clinical nursing situation in which you were involved. Write your description of the situation, and then apply the rest of Gibbs' model to reflect on the situation.

## Reflective writing – keeping a journal or reflective diary

The purpose of reflective writing is to support the process of reflection while, at the same time, providing evidence of learning (Hurford, 2009). Many people find it takes time to develop reflective skills, so it is important to build on this early in your course (Cottrell, 2008). Reflective writing requires a commitment of time and energy as it involves looking at a situation in depth, but it is an excellent basis for professional development, both as a student and when you become a registered nurse. The reasons why writing, rather than thinking or verbalising, are beneficial are that writing:

- is an active process;

- organises and encourages deep thoughts and feelings;

- enables the gaining of more control over thoughts, emotions, responses and behaviour;

- encourages self-awareness, self-diagnosis and honesty;

- encourages examination of the negative, development of the positive and can reveal uncertainties which need exploring;

- is done for the purpose of learning;

- provides a way of exploring a range of issues from different perspectives;

- stimulates change.

(Jasper, 2006; Kitson, 2005; Cottrell, 2003)

Records of reflection over time should be kept in a portfolio as evidence of professional development and contribute to your personal development plan. This is essential for registered nurses, but it is also expected of, and is good practice for students. It allows you to look for themes that recur and perhaps are not resolved, or conflicts that present themselves in a variety of forms. It also provides a safe base for you to explore your feelings which can be challenging as you may discover truths about yourself which are embarrassing or make you feel uncomfortable. For this reason, Burns and Bulman (2000) suggest journals should be kept private and only selected aspects made available for more public reading.

Any of the frameworks already mentioned in this chapter can be used to write reflectively, or if you prefer you can write using 'free-flowing' text. As you become used to this process you will develop confidence in your own evaluation and judgement of your work. The important aspect is that *you* are writing about *your* experiences, so you should write in the first person. Focus on yourself, but avoid using reflection as a way of blaming or taking out anger on others; it is your own role you need to consider and how you would make a similar situation more manageable next time. Openness, honesty and critical analysis are the key features you need to consider, along with identification of any actions required in terms of your development.

Reflection is not all about 'clinical incidents'. You can reflect on your course by focusing on your development and progress as a whole, both academically and clinically. Cottrell (2008) suggests you consider:

- your feelings about your course, the lecturers, other students, your progress;

- things you find difficult – challenges;

- changes in your attitude or motivation;

- how you tackle tasks – your strategies;

- things you find out about yourself;

- thoughts about how you learn best;

- ideas that arise from your studies;

- how different areas of studies link up;

- how your studies relate to real life.

These aspects can act as a basis for discussion with your tutors, along with any possible options you may have to address any issues arising from your reflection.

## ACTIVITY 9.2

Using a different model from Gibbs', write a short reflective account of a recent situation you encountered while studying at university (not a clinical event). Compare the reflective model used with Gibbs' model and consider which one you found the most useful.

# Professional development

The following topics – portfolios and profiles and clinical supervision – give a brief outline of what is expected of you when you register as a nurse with the NMC. They all involve reflection and are therefore discussed briefly in the following pages.

## Portfolios and profiles

The demonstration of professional competence is a crucial element of being a registered, accountable practitioner (Jasper, 2006). The NMC states that all registered nurses are required to create and maintain a portfolio, and within that, a personal professional profile demonstrating fitness to remain eligible to practice. It should outline career progression and identify learning opportunities for the future.

You may or may not be familiar with the concept of maintaining your own portfolio, but, on the whole, any portfolio you may be required to compile as a student will ask you to provide evidence according to pre-specified criteria (achievement of competences and learning outcomes, etc.). Post-registration portfolios have a different focus as they require evidence to demonstrate fitness for continuing practice. However, there is sometimes confusion as to what a profile is and what a portfolio is, so Brown (1995) offers the following definitions:

### Portfolio

'A private collection of evidence which demonstrates the continuing acquisition of skills, knowledge, attitudes, understanding and achievements. It is both retrospective and prospective, as well as reflecting the current stage of development and activity of the individual' (Brown, 1995, p. 2).

### Profile

'A collection of evidence which is selected from your portfolio for a particular purpose, and for the attention of a particular audience. Therefore an array of profiles can be developed to meet different needs; for example, when applying for a job, for professional development review, etc' (Brown, 1995, p. 5).

Jasper (2006, p. 155) suggests that Brown's definitions emphasise several features.

- Their individual nature: portfolios are unique to the person compiling them and provide a permanent record of that person's professional history.

- They are 'dynamic' in nature, in that they reflect the past but anticipate and plan for the future.

- They document and record specific 'attributes' of the individual concerned.

- They comprise various types of 'evidence'.

The NMC states that a profile is:

> a record of career progress and professional development. It is not a CV, a daily diary of events or your whole life history! A profile is a flexible but comprehensive account of your professional development. However, it is more than a record of achievement. It is based on a regular process of reflection and recording what you learn from every day experiences, as well as planned learning activity. Your profile

is your personal document. It does not belong to the NMC or your employer and its contents are private and confidential to you.

(www.nmc-uk.org)

(Although an NMC definition, the last sentence can sound a bit confusing as it is your *portfolio* which is private and confidential to you – you will be asked to share sections of it (i.e. your profile) with others).

Jasper (2006) highlights the benefits of maintaining a portfolio as helping you to:

- assess your current standards of practice;

- develop your analytical skills through reflection on what you do;

- review and evaluate past experience and learning to help you plan for the future;

- provide effective and current information if you apply for a job or a course;

- demonstrate experiential learning which may allow you to obtain credit towards further qualifications.

### *Organising and documenting your information*

There is no approved format for a portfolio or the profile sections within it. Whatever format you choose - ring binder, box file, memory stick or one of the profiles available commercially – the main factors should be flexibility, accessibility and confidentiality. Your portfolio will contain personal information, so it should not be accessible to others without your permission. At the same time, you should not document any information which could identify patients, clients or carers as this could constitute a breach of confidentiality. For these reasons, you could consider dividing your portfolio into two sections: one containing confidential information (such as reflections, etc.) and the other containing material that the NMC may require for audit purposes – see the NMC *Prep Handbook* (2011) regarding audit.

As there is no definite format as to what should be included in a portfolio, because it is personal to you, you might wish to consider the following as a guide:

- personal details – CV and employment record;

- educational and academic record;

- personal and professional development (past and present);

- professional work with key learning points;

- reflective reviews with key learning points and an action plan;

- critical incident analysis;

- copies of articles written, or other written publications;

- non-nursing experiences;

- future development and career aspirations.

Boud *et al.* (1985) give guidelines and tips on how to develop and maintain a portfolio which may be of help.

- Seek out a method which suits you – it is important to keep your portfolio personal. Write about what it is important for you, not what others say you should;

- Be frank, honest and spontaneous in your entries – use your own words, say what you feel;

- Have a positive approach when writing – write regularly and stick at it;

- Feel free to express yourself in diagrams, pictures or other types of material;

- A portfolio is meant to be a workbook – work through entries a number of times, go back to early entries and further reflect on them;

- Focus on things that are important – do not waste time on trivialities;

- Do not be rigid in the way you keep your portfolio – be prepared to change your methods;

- Record experiences as soon as possible after they happen, and in as much detail as possible;

- Important issues may need to be shared with others, and you should record feedback – this will deepen your understanding of situations.

(adapted from Boud *et al.*, 1985)

### Clinical supervision

Clinical supervision is a term that has been used by registered nurses and other health care professionals to provide a purposeful, practice-focused relationship that enables the nurse to reflect on their practice with the support of a skilled supervisor (Peate, 2006). It was introduced in the workplace for nurses during the 1990s, following the Department of Health's document *Vision for the Future* (Department of Health, 1993) as a way of using reflective practice and shared experiences as part of continuing professional development (CPD). The concept, however, has been long established in professions such as midwifery, social work, psychotherapy and counselling.

The NMC (2008, p. 1) believes that 'essentially, clinical supervision allows a registered nurse to receive professional supervision in the workplace by a skilled supervisor. It allows nurses and midwives to develop their skills and knowledge and helps them to improve care'.

Clinical supervision also has the support of the RCN (2003), which states that it enables registered nurses to:

- reflect on nursing practice;

- identify solutions to problems;

- increase understanding of professional issues;

- improve standards of patient care;

- further develop their skills and knowledge;

- enhance understanding of their own practice;

- identify room for improvement;

- devise new ways of learning;

- gain professional support.

Clinical supervision is different from any discussion you may have with your line manager when you are registered, in that it involves stepping back and reflecting on practice with a clinical supervisor who is external to your immediate workplace. It should not be confused with appraisal, development review or any other management activity. It is not currently a mandatory requirement from the NMC, and anything said in sessions should be confidential.

The clinical supervision sessions themselves should be carefully structured and managed with clearly defined aims and objectives. Ground rules and responsibilities should be clearly defined and there should be a contract of commitment from both supervisor and supervisees in order for it to be a meaningful exercise.

There are various models or approaches to clinical supervision; one-to-one supervision, group supervision, or peer group supervision. The choice of approach will depend on a number of factors, including personal choice, access to supervision, length of experience, qualifications, availability of supervisory groups, etc. However, everyone participating in clinical supervision will have a supervisor who is a skilled professional and assists other practitioners in the development of their skills, knowledge and professional values.

Fitzgerald (2000, p. 155) believes that:

> within these types of supervisory relationships reflection plays an important role in the clinical supervision process. The use of a reflective framework facilitates a structured approach to the agenda of the supervisory meeting and helps maintain the focus on practice whilst enabling a questioning approach.

Driscoll (1994) agrees but suggests that not all reflective practice is clinical supervision but all good supervision is potentially reflective practice. He also points out that clinical supervision is not only about reflecting on the big issues surrounding clinical practice, but also on the seemingly insignificant and most ordinary of practice activities.

Driscoll's (2000) model of clinical supervision is probably the most widely known and used. It is in the form of reflective practice, but the essential difference is that it involves another person helping someone to reflect. It is cyclical in nature and is known as the WHAT? It contains three elements, these elements being used for a supervisee to prepare for clinical supervision.

* WHAT? – a description of the event;

* So WHAT? – an analysis of the event;

* Now WHAT? – proposed actions following the event.

Driscoll (2000, p. 30) also lists a number of trigger questions, which are not dissimilar to those posed by Johns (2010) and Stephenson (1993, cited in Palmer *et al.*, 1994), but in addition he lists some skills and attributes required (of both supervisor and supervisee) for effective clinical supervision. They are:

* a willingness to learn from what happens in practice;

* being open enough to share elements of practice with other people;

- being motivated enough to replay aspects of clinical practice;

- having knowledge for clinical practice, which can emerge from within, as well as outside clinical practice;

- being aware of the conditions necessary for reflection to occur;

- a belief that it is possible to change as a practitioner;

- the ability to describe in detail before analysing practice problems;

- recognising the consequences of reflection;

- the ability to articulate what happens in practice;

- a belief that there is no end point about learning in practice;

- not being defensive about what other people notice about one's practice;

- being courageous enough to act on reflection;

- working out schemes to personally action what has been learned;

- being honest in describing clinical practice to others.

## Chapter summary

- Reflection is an important learning strategy and encourages life-long learning.

- Good reflective practice underpins good professional practice.

- There are many different models for reflection and no one is better than another.

- Reflection is personal but you may be asked to share your experiences with others.

- Once registered, you will be expected to keep a portfolio of your experiences (NMC, 2011).

## References

Boud, D., Keogh, R. & Walkwe, D. (1985) *Reflection: Turning Experience into Learning*. London: Kogan Page.

Brown, R. (1995) *Portfolio Development and Profiling for Nurses* (2nd edition). Central Health Studies series No 3. (series editor John Tingle). Lancaster: Quay Publishing.

Burns, S. & Bulman, C. (2000) *The Reflective Practice in Nursing*. Oxford: Blackwell Science.

Cottrell, S. (2003) *Skills for Success*. New York: Palgrave Macmillan.

Cottrell, S. (2008) *The Study Skills Handbook* (3rd edition). New York: Palgrave Macmillan.

Department of Health (1993) *A Vision for the Future: The Nursing, Midwifery and Health Visiting Contribution to Health and Health Care*. London: HMSO.

Dewey, J. (1938) *Experience and Education*. New York: Macmillan, in: Jasper, M. (2006) *Professional Development, Reflection and Decision-Making*. Oxford: Blackwell Publishing.

Driscoll, J. (1994) Reflective practice for practice. *Senior Nurse*, **14(1)**: 47–50.

Driscoll, J. (2000) *Practising Clinical Supervision*. London: Bailliere Tindall.

Fitzgerald, M. (2000) *Clinical Supervision and Reflective Practice* in: Bulman, C. & Burns, S. (ed.) *Reflective Practice in Nursing* (2nd edition, Ch 5). Oxford: Blackwell Scientific.

Gibbs, G. (1998) *Learning by Doing: A Guide to Teaching and Learning Methods*. London: Further Education Unit.

Hurford, A. (2009) http://pd.nottingham.ac.uk/eng/Learning-Teaching/ (accessed 20 November 2012)

Jasper, M. (2006) *Professional Development, Reflection and Decision-Making*. Oxford: Blackwell Publishing.

Johns, C. (2006) *Engaging Reflection in Practice: A Narrative Approach*. Oxford: Blackwell Publishing.

Johns, C. (2010) *Guided Reflection* (2nd edition). Oxford: Wiley-Blackwell.

Kitson, K. (2005) www.ibms.org (accessed 20 November 2012)

Moon, J. (2004) *A Handbook of Reflective and Experiential Learning*. London: Routledge.

Nursing and Midwifery Council (2008) *Clinical Supervision* (advice sheet). London: NMC.

Nursing and Midwifery Council (2011) *The Prep Handbook*. London: NMC.

Palmer, A., Burns, S. & Bulman, C. (eds) (1994) *Reflective Practice in Nursing. The Growth of the Professional Practitioner*. Oxford: Blackwell.

Peate, I. (2006) *Becoming a Nurse in the 21st Century*. Chichester: John Wiley.

Price, B. (2002) Effective learning No. 3: Reflective observations in practice. *Nursing Standard*, **17(9):** S1–2.

Royal College of Nursing (2003) *Clinical Supervision in the Workplace: Guidance for Occupational Health Nurses*. London: RCN.

Somerset Academy (2005) *Reflective Framework*. Somerset Academy.

Stephenson, S (1993) *Reflection – a Student Perspective* in Palmer, A., Burns, S. & Bulman, C. (ed.) (1994) *Reflective Practice in Nursing. The Growth of the Professional Practitioner*. Oxford: Blackwell.

Whitehead, E. & Mason, T. (2007) *Study Skills for Nurses*. London: Sage.

# 10
# STUDY SKILLS AND INFORMATION TECHNOLOGY

The aim of this chapter is to provide a brief overview of some of the key factors associated with study skills and using information technology (IT).

| **Learning Outcomes** | • identify, discuss and make use of some key study skills; |
|---|---|
| On completion of this chapter you should be able to: | • make use of some key skills for researching information online. |

## Study skills

The term 'study' can be defined as 'the application of the mind to the acquisition of knowledge' (www.dictionary.reference.com). Most of us probably never really think about the skills required for studying – we just get on and do it. However, it is suggested that the more study skills and strategies you apply and practise, the more independent and confident you can become in any learning situation (www.itscotland.org.uk). It should also be remembered that no two people study in exactly the same way, so what works for one person may well not work for another. The following section offers some widely recognised skills that you might like to try, to see if they work for you.

## Reading

When you start a nursing course, you will have the same problem as every other student – how to get through the vast amount of reading you are required to do in order to complete the programme. There will not be enough time to read everything line by line so you will have to learn the skills that enable you to read efficiently and effectively within the time you have available. The following provides a brief overview of some of the main skills involved.

### Environment

Before we look at reading skills, think about the environment in which you are reading. It is most unlikely that you will be able to concentrate on reading and understanding if you are in an environment that is noisy and uncomfortable. Try to find a physical environment that is conducive for you to read in, for example by turning off the television or moving into a quiet room, or using a library. Other things you might consider include making sure the lighting is adequate, and that you are comfortably seated and working at a table if you are going to take notes. Work out what time of the day is best for you to study, and read at this time whenever possible. Try to avoid important reading if you are tired or if your eyes ache.

### Styles or types of reading

Your style of reading should be chosen to suit the task. Styles or types of reading include the following:

Skimming

This is the technique you may use when you are going through a newspaper or magazine. The idea is that you read quickly to get the main points, and skip over the detail. It's also useful to skim when reading academic text to:

- preview a passage before you read it in detail;
- refresh your understanding of a passage after you have read it in detail;
- decide if a book in the library or bookshop is right for you – to do this look at the title, author, synopsis (on back cover or front flap), contents page and date of publication for an indication of its relevance to your needs.

Scanning

Having decided on the potential usefulness of a book from your skim, you need then to confirm that it will indeed be useful to you for your studies. This involves a more in-depth examination or scanning of a text for specific information relevant to your task or topic area. This can include scanning:

- the synopsis on the back cover of the book;
- the introduction or preface of a book;
- the first or last paragraphs of chapters;
- the concluding chapter of a book.

Detailed reading

This is where you read sections and chapters in full, identifying and extracting the main points or examples from the text.

Critical reading

Critical reading requires you to evaluate the information and arguments in the text. You need to distinguish fact from opinion, and look at arguments given for and against the various issues. This is also where, having read appropriately more than one text on a similar topic, you begin to identify and compare and contrast any bias, objectivity and perspective that they may have. Using such comparisons when writing an essay can help you to produce a balanced and objective piece of work.

## *Reading skills*

Active reading

When you are reading for your course, in order to help maintain your concentration and understanding, you will need to make sure you are as actively involved with the text as possible. Active reading can include a variety of techniques:

- **Underlining and highlighting** – pick out what you think are the most important parts of what you are reading. If you are a visual learner, you will find it helpful to use different colours to highlight different aspects of what you are reading. (NB: Only do this with your own copy of texts or on photocopies, not with books or journals borrowed from the library, or from fellow students or lecturers).

- **Note key words** – record the main headings as you read. Use one or two keywords for each point. When you do not want to mark the text, keep a folder of notes you make whilst reading.

SQ3R method

One well-recognised model of active reading that incorporates some of these suggestions is the SQ3R method. The SQ3R method involves five steps which should, if followed, help you to get the most out of your reading. The five steps are:
1. survey;
2. question;
3. read;

4.  recall / recite;
5.  review.

- **S = Survey** – This first step helps you to focus on the author's topic and purpose (what is he/she trying to get across to the reader?) and on main ideas in the text. Before reading, you need to survey the material. This can involve looking briefly at the title of the chapter, any boldface headings or subheadings, any visual aids to points such as charts, maps, and diagrams, and reading the chapter introduction and summary. Only a few minutes need be spent surveying the text to ease you into the reading.

- **Q = Question** – This step requires deliberate effort. The key here is to develop a questioning attitude as you read the chapter or text. This can be achieved by, for example, turning the title, headings and/ or subheadings into questions (e.g. if the subheading is 'recording references' your question may be 'why do I need to record references?'). It can also include looking at any questions that might be posed by the author through set activities or at the end of the chapter. Writing the questions down keeps you alert and helps focus your concentration on what you need to learn from your reading.

- **R = Read** – For this step you need to read the material actively and try to answer any of the questions you have raised. Note down and answer questions in your own words, as this will enable you to understand and comprehend more fully the text you are reading. Look for the main ideas and important details, notice italicised or bold words, study any visual aids and make sure you understand their meaning and relevance to the text. Reduce your reading speed for difficult passages of text, and stop and re-read parts that are not clear.

- **R = Recite or recall** – Keep challenging yourself to make sure you have an understanding of what you are reading by recitation and constant recall. After each section, stop and think back to your questions. See if you can answer them from memory. If not, take a look back at the text. Try to recall main headings, important issues and concepts in your own words and what graphs and charts indicate. Do this as often as you need, as it can help you learn and apply the knowledge to other areas.

- **R = Review** – The review is an assessment of what you have accomplished. When you have finished a chapter, an article, etc., go back over the questions you posed during your reading. See if you can still answer them. If not, look back and refresh your memory; re-read if necessary. The review is a good time to go over any notes you have taken to help clarify points you may have missed or don't understand. It can also be useful to make flash cards for important points or for those questions that you found difficult to answer. The best time to review is when you have just finished studying.

(www.bized.co.uk; www.adprima.com; www.uefap.com; openlearn.open.ac.uk; www.gre.ac.uk)

## Taking notes

Note-taking is a skill that you will need to use many times as a student of nursing. Effective note-taking should have a purpose and be well organised, and can be a time-saving skill. By making notes you actively process and interpret ideas and information; this aids concentration and understanding and should enable you to learn more. Notes can also play an important part in planning assignments and projects by helping you identify the main points and organise your ideas into a logical order. When preparing for an exam, notes can provide a concise record of information for you to revise from. There is no one 'correct' way to take notes. Everyone tends to develop their own way of taking notes, and very different approaches can be equally effective.

The following are tips on how you might become an efficient and successful note-taker. These can apply equally to taking notes from a verbal presentation or from a written text.

### Amount

The whole point of note-taking is to be able to summarise information in a different, shorter form to use later. Whichever strategy you use, it is important to realise you do not have to copy down everything you read or hear. If you do, note-taking will just become time-consuming, ineffective and a boring and passive way of learning.

### Key words and phrases

When making notes, listen or look out for key words and phrases such as 'the most important factor is'. In your notes, key words and phrases should trigger your memory or lead on to other ideas or explanations, so they must be easy to find when you are reviewing your notes at a later date. This may be achieved by:

- underlining important points once, very important points twice;

- using capital letters;

- drawing boxes around the keywords;

- drawing an asterisk (*) next to the main idea;

- going over the most important points with a highlighter pen;

- using different coloured inks for different themes or approaches.

### Symbols and abbreviations

When you take notes, particularly in a lecture, seminar, etc., or even on clinical placement, you will rarely have time to write in full sentences, or sometimes even full words. It is therefore useful to develop your own set of symbols and abbreviations. Some of the more common ones, which you will probably already be aware of, include:

| | |
|---|---|
| e.g. | for example |
| i.e. | that is |
| + | and/plus |
| = | equals |
| NB | note well |
| % | percentage |
| etc. | and so on |
| < | less than |
| > | greater than |
| ∴ | therefore |
| a/c | account |
| no. | number |
| ref. | reference |
| vs | against/as opposed to |
| w/ | with |
| w/o | without |

Remember though – do keep a copy of any of your own abbreviations in the front of your notes file so that you can remember them at a later date.

### Mind mapping (spray diagram / spider diagram)

Mind maps offer a non-linear and diagrammatical way to organise key ideas from your lectures, seminars and reading. They also have the potential to present a large amount of information on one page and act as a summary for more detailed notes.

In a mind map the main topic or argument is placed at the centre of the page (see *Figure 10.1*).

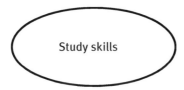

*Figure 10.1 – Main topic of the mind map*

Ideas that relate to the main topic are then placed on branches that directly connect to the central topic (see *Figure 10.2*).

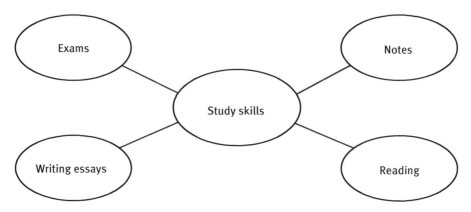

*Figure 10.2 – Main branches of the main map*

Each of these main ideas then develops its own branches of ideas (see *Figure 10.3*).

As each theme is developed you add branch lines from each topic. Sometimes, it can also help to add colours and/or differently shaped boxes.

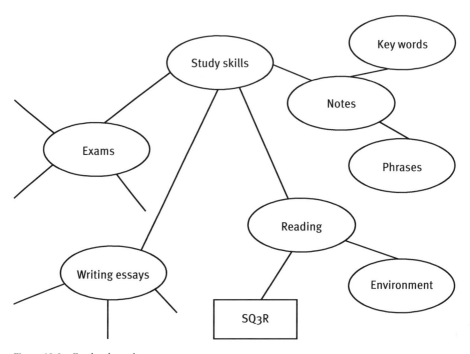

*Figure 10.3 – Further branches*

Once complete, and you have all your ideas down on paper, look for links between themes and indicate them with an arrow or chain. When using this technique for an assignment, exam, etc. it can be useful to number each theme to show the order in which you are going to refer to them.

### Handwriting, spelling and grammar

When you have completed a set of notes, check back and make sure that you can actually understand the notes you have made and that your handwriting has not become unreadable. Make any alterations while the topic is still fresh in your mind or when there are people who can clarify what you should have written. As long as your meaning is clear don't worry about your spelling and grammar. At this stage it is better to focus on recording the information, so achieving perfection in spelling and grammar is not important – save this for your assignment or exam.

### Plagiarism and paraphrasing

Plagiarism can become an issue, especially when taking notes from written texts. In order to avoid this, do not just copy down material verbatim from another source without putting it in quotation marks and noting its origin – always put the full reference and page number in the margin beside the quote. If you do not do this, you may well forget that these words are not your own. If you then include them as your own in an assignment, report, etc., you will have committed plagiarism. It is better when taking notes to paraphrase (i.e. put a passage into your own words) wherever possible. However, you will still need to acknowledge the initial source of your information in your essay, etc. If you do this at the note-taking stage, there can be no confusion later on.

### *Organise your notes*

Although it seems to be common sense, it is surprising how many people do not organise effectively the notes they take during their course of study. It is important to have a good system for organising and storing your notes, as doing this well will save you a great deal of time when it comes to using them when preparing for an assignment or exam. Whatever system you decide to use or develop, it should suit your personal needs. The following are some suggestions as to how your notes may be organised effectively.

- Use a separate file for each subject area.

- Use file dividers to separate major topics.

- Arrange notes under headings or questions.

- Number and label pages so that you can re-file them easily.

- Use one lecture note book per subject.

- Always leave a margin down one side of the page for future notes, references, comments, etc.

> (Northledge, 2007; www.uefap.com; openlearn.open.ac.uk; mail.baylorschool.org; www.mindtools.com; www.litemind.com)

## Writing essays

Writing essays is something that you will have to do on a regular basis in order to demonstrate your understanding of a topic in a well-structured written format. There is, once again, no single correct way to approach essay writing; you need to find what approach suits you best. The following section offers some tips to support or develop your approach.

### Understanding the question

The basis of any essay should always begin from an understanding of what you are trying to achieve. It is therefore important to make sure that you know exactly what is required of you before you begin to research or to draft your essay. If you have been given a specific question, you need to begin by 'unpicking' the information it contains. This can be done by carefully examining the words of the question, looking for: the **content words** that indicate the subject matter with which the essay should deal; **limiting words** that specify the particular aspect or aspects of the subject on which the essay should focus; and the **instruction words** which tell you how to approach the topic.

Essay questions usually contain one or more of the following key words that indicate what you are being asked to do.

- **Account for**: give reasons for, explain how something came about, clarify.

- **Assess**: decide the importance / value of something and give reasons.

- **Analyse**: examine in detail, consider the various parts of the whole and describe the interrelationship between them.

- **Comment on**: explain the importance of.

- **Compare**: examine the objects in question with a view to demonstrating their similarities.

- **Contrast**: examine the objects in question for the purpose of demonstrating differences, or examine two or more opposing ideas or arguments to highlight their differences.

- **Define**: state precisely the meaning of something using example – a simple statement is often not enough, it needs to be explored in detail.

- **Discuss**: explain and give different views about something – this can include your own views as long as they are based on sound evidence (i.e. they are referenced).

- **Examine**: look at very carefully.

- **Explain**: make very clear why something is the way it is, or why it happens.

- **Evaluate**: examine the evidence and decide the value of something, make a judgement about it, based on sound evidence.

- **Give an acount of**: describe in detail how something happened.

- **Illustrate**: make something very clear, using evidence and examples.

- **Outline**: give a short description of the main points.

- **Justify**: support a particular idea, using evidence, and show why particular conclusions were made – include counter-arguments.

- **Show**: make clear, demonstrate evidence for.

- **Summarise**: outline the main points briefly.

### Essay planning

Once you have decided what is required, researched the topic and read through your notes, you should then make an essay plan. Time spent on essay planning is rarely time wasted as it provides an opportunity to identify the main themes, sections or areas and how all the various pieces of information fit together. An essay plan is also useful to take to a tutorial so that you can discuss with your tutor your ideas about completing the assignment. The plan should be written in a way that works for you personally, for example as a mind map, linear notes or a set of boxes, etc.

### Structure of an essay

The structure of the essay is important because it demonstrates that you are able to order your thoughts in a systematic, logical way and provides a sense of direction through the essay. The accepted basic framework for any essay is:

- introduction;

- main text/body;

- conclusion.

The introduction

The purpose of the introduction should be to set the context and direction of the essay. It should therefore:

- be clear that it is an introduction;

- if required, set the question topic against a wider background (set the context);

- identify and/or define any key terms;

- briefly summarise the overall theme of the essay, indicating the main points to be made and, possibly, the order in which they are to be presented – that is, explain what the essay is going to do.

## Main body / text

The main body of the text is where the main ideas or arguments are developed. Depending on the length of the essay, it will contain several sections, each divided into paragraphs. The paragraphs should be logically linked as you develop the themes or ideas. In the main body you should:

- present key points clearly;

- present ideas or arguments backed up by evidence from your reading;

- accurately cite quotations and references to other works;

- label any diagrams, figures or tables correctly.

## Conclusion

The conclusion should follow logically from, and be based on, what you have presented in the main body of your essay as it brings together the main ideas explored. This can be achieved by:

- briefly summarising the main ideas and arguments;

- linking back to to the title / topic showing how you have answered the question or drawn a relevant conclusion;

- making clear why conclusions reached are important or significant;

- not including any new ideas.

## *Referencing*

Referencing is the standardised method of acknowledging sources of information. When writing an essay, report or dissertation, it is usual to make reference (i.e. to identify the place where the original citation can be found) to the sources that you have used, referred to, or taken quotes from. These references might be from, for example, journals, newspaper articles, books or book chapters, government reports, internet publications. When you refer to someone else's work or directly quote from it, you must refer to the author / editor both in the text and in a reference list or bibliography at the end of your work. Citing accurate references in academic work is important for the following reasons:

- to give credit to other authors' concepts and ideas;

- to provide evidence of the extent of your reading;

- to allow a reader to locate the cited references easily;

- to avoid being accused of plagiarism.

Plagiarism can be defined as: 'the action or practice of taking someone else's work, idea, etc. and passing it off as one's own' (Oxford English Dictionary, 2012, p. 1621). This is a potentially serious offence in an academic environment, but it can easily be avoided by acknowledging all sources of information. Failure to do this could result in work being downgraded or even unmarked. The reference list should contain details of all the sources you have mentioned in your essay. A bibliography contains sources you have consulted but not mentioned in your essay. You may be asked for just a reference list or you may be asked for both references and a bibliography. You need to check your assignment guidelines to see what is required.

There are many systems for the citation of references, and you should follow the system that will be identified in your course handbook or assessment guidelines. The most commonly used systems in the UK are the Harvard system and Vancouver system.

### Harvard system

The Harvard system cites the author's surname and year of publication in the text, e.g. (Jones, 2004), and provides a reference list of any text citations in alphabetical order by author at the end of the assignment. It is here that additional details are noted, such as surname and initials, the title of the article, book or chapter, place of publication and the publisher.

### Vancouver system

In the Vancouver system, a number is assigned to each reference as it is used. Even if the author is named in the text, a number must still be used. The original number assigned to the reference is used each time that reference is cited in the text. The first reference cited will be numbered 1 in the text, and the second reference cited will be numbered 2, and so on. If a reference cited number 1 is used again later in the text, it should be cited using the number 1 again. References are listed in numerical order in a reference list / bibliography at the end of the essay.

## *A few final points about essays*

### Style of writing

Precision of language is very important. Ensure that your writing style:

- uses complete, straightforward sentences that are varied, not too simple or too convoluted (complex sentences do not necessarily signify complex thought), and also avoids writing in note form;
- avoids using slang and colloquialisms;
- only quotes relevant material and does not overuse quotes (it is much better to interpret information in your own words);
- does not use inappropriate analogies;
- does not adopt a subjective or emotive tone;
- does not make assertions or sweeping statements without supporting evidence or argument;
- is not repetitive.

### Paragraphs

There should be one main theme per paragraph and you should use paragraphs to signal the natural breaks in your argument when the focus of attention shifts. Excessively long paragraphs should be avoided and, where possible, the first sentence of each paragraph should link in some way to the previous paragraph. This allows for the flow or continuity of argument which is a very important quality in essays.

### Link words

Link words are words that provide 'signposts' along the way, which help identify connections and relationships between key ideas. They include:

- words that lead the reader forwards, such as 'again', 'furthermore', 'finally';
- words that make the reader stop and compare, such as 'however', 'although', 'nonetheless';
- words that develop and summarise, such as 'clearly', 'therefore', 'in conclusion'.

Length

The length of any assignment will be identified in the assignment guidelines. It is important that you are as close to your word limit as possible, as most universities or colleges will probably have clearly identified mark penalties if the word count of an assignment is more than 10 per cent over or under the stated amount for that piece of work. Usually it will be requested that you record your word count at the end of the assignment, and again failure to do so might result in the loss of some marks.

Proofread

The final preparation of the essay for submission is important. This includes carefully proofreading your essay, or asking a friend or relative to do this for you. Even better is getting someone to read your work back to you. Notice any faults of grammar and make sure you correct them before submitting the work. Spelling errors can sometimes be more difficult to detect, simply because you may not know how a particular word is spelt. Nevertheless, you should try to correct as many spelling errors as possible. Most word-processing packages include both spelling and grammar checks – use both but don't rely on them completely as some words may be spelt correctly but used in the wrong context such as, for example, 'write' and 'right'.

Presentation

Print out your work in hard copy, preferably using double spacing or 1.5 spacing when word-processing and include wide margins (both make the text far easier to read and comment upon).

Don't forget to keep at least one copy of your assignment; they can occasionally get lost in the system.
(Northledge, 2007; www.bolton.ac.uk/; www.staffs.ac.uk; www.napier.ac.uk; www.theory.org.uk/; www.bized.co.uk; www.shef.ac.uk; www.soton.ac.uk)

## Using information technology (IT)

Information technology has significantly changed the way ideas and information are recorded and communicated in all areas of life, including the study and practice of nursing. According to Northledge (2007, pp. 51–52) computers help with studies in several different ways:

- researching online;

- making notes;

- managing your studies – helping to organise and keep track of studies;

- word-processing;

- working with numbers and charts – computer software can be perfect for creating tables, charts and graphs;

- storing information;

- talking online;

- e-learning.

It is beyond the scope of this section to explore all of the above in any depth. However, a few tips are offered for researching online and the issue of e-learning will be explored a little further.

### Researching online

Some general tips include the following.

Narrow your research topic

The internet allows access to so much information that you can easily be overwhelmed. Before you start your search, think about what you're looking for and, if possible, formulate some very specific questions to direct and limit your search. Try not to use broad or general terms – rather, use terms that are more specific to the topic you are researching. You can also sometimes narrow your search by looking at sites that you may have previously used and that are relevant to your topic.

Boolean operators

Boolean operators are words that allow you to combine search terms and can be utilised in most search engines. The three most common are '**and**', '**or**' and '**not**'.

- **and** – narrows the search and retrieves sites/records containing all the words it separates. For example, entering 'values AND ethics' would instruct the search engine to find web pages that contain both words, 'values' and 'ethics'.

- **or** – broadens the search and retrieves sites / records containing any of the words it separates. For example, entering 'values OR ethics' would cause the search engine to look for web pages that contain either the word 'values' or the word 'ethics', but not necessarily both words. You need to be mindful that this could result in the return of thousands or even millions of sites. 'Or' is most useful when the same term may appear in two different ways like, for example, using 'evidence-based practice OR EBP' to find information about evidence-based practice.

- **not** – narrows the search and retrieves sites that do not contain the term following the 'not' – i.e. it finds the first word but not the second. This limitation is helpful when you know your search term is likely to appear with another term that does not interest you, for example 'toddler NOT baby'.

## Exact phrases

If you want your search engine to search for an exact phrase, put quotation marks around the phrase.

## Include appropriate alternative or synonymous terms

Scan the titles and abstracts of the sites / records you find for other possible keywords or synonyms you may not have thought of using. For example, a search on the common name 'St John's wort' finds records which include the Latin name *hypericum* and the extract name 'hypericin'. A good revised search strategy would be: 'St John's wort OR hypericum OR hypericin'.

## Know your search engines and subject directories

Search engines (e.g. Google, Yahoo and AltaVista) can differ considerably in how they work, how much of the internet they search, and the kind of results you can expect to get from them. Spending some time learning what each search engine will do and how best to use it can help you avoid a lot of frustration and wasted time later. There are a great many good academic resources available on the internet, including hundreds of online journals and sites set up by universities and scholarly or nursing organisations. The following are some core bibliographic e–resources.

- The BNI (British Nursing Index) provides reference to journals and articles, some conference papers and major reports on aspects of education and nursing from the UK and some English language international publications.

- CINAHL (Cumulative Index to Nursing and Allied Health Literature) has international coverage and indexes over 1600 nursing and allied health journals.

- CRD (Centre for Reviews and Dissemination) enables the search of the Database of Abstracts of Reviews of Effects (DARE), the NHS Economic Evaluation Database (NHSEED) and the Health Technology Assessment database (HTA).

- The Cochrane Library is designed to provide evidence to inform health care decision-making.

- MEDLINE (Medical Literature Analysis and Retrieval System Online), ASSIA (Applied Social Science Index and Abstracts), IBSS (International Bibliography of the Social Sciences).

Evaluate the information

If you are not using recognised academic resources such as those above, you need to remember that anyone can put whatever they want on a website; there is no review or screening process, and there are no agreed standard ways of identifying subjects and creating cross-references. Therefore you must always think critically about the information you have found on the internet. Some of the questions you should be asking yourself are:

- who is the author?

- who is sponsoring the website?

- what is the audience level?

- is the information current and up to date?

- is the content reliable and accurate?

Remember that if you decide to use the information, you are responsible for ensuring that it is reliable and accurate.

(See also *Chapter 7* on 'Evidence-based practice' for hints on how to review articles.)

Keep a detailed record of sites you visit and the sites you use

Doing research on the internet inevitably means visiting some sites that are useful and many that are not. Keeping a record of useful websites is good practice so that you can revisit them at a later date. Also, if you are using the information in an essay or an assignment you can acknowledge the source of that information easily and accurately. Using the browser's history function for this is not really good practice as it will retain the web addresses or URLs of all the sites you visit, good or bad. In addition, if you are using a computer at your place of study, the memory in the history file may be erased at the end of your session. It is much better either to note down accurately on paper or to bookmark the sites you've found useful, so that you will have a permanent record.

### Double-check all URLs that you put in your paper

It is easy to make mistakes with complicated internet addresses, and typing errors will invalidate your references. If you type them into the location box of your browser you will be able to check that you have the correct address because it will take you to the correct site.

(Northledge, 2007; www.uleth.ca; jerz.setonhill.edu; www3.northern.edu)

## *Electronic learning (e-learning)*

E-learning is a unifying term used to describe the learning and delivery of a training or education programme using a computer or electronic device (for example, a mobile phone). Its use has steadily increased within nursing programmes both at pre- and post-registration levels.

Some other terms frequently interchanged with 'e-learning' include:

- online learning;
- online education;
- distance education;
- distance learning;
- technology-based training;
- web-based training;
- computer-based training (generally thought of as learning from a CD-ROM).

### Types of e-learning

E-learning comes in many variations and is often a combination of the following:

- purely online – no face-to-face meetings;
- blended learning – combination of online and face-to-face;

- synchronous – live interaction between tutor and students. Students log in at a specific time and for a specified duration;

- asynchronous – students learn through internet-based, network-based or stored disk-based modules. Interaction with others includes via e-mail, online discussion groups and online bulletin boards;

- teacher-led group;

- self-study;

- web-based study;

- computer-based (CD-ROM) study;

- video / audio tape.

## Features and benefits of e-learning

Wherever you look in the literature it is clear that the use of e-learning can demonstrate significant benefits. These benefits are that:

- learning is self-paced and provides the learner with a chance to speed up or slow down as necessary;

- learning is self-directed, thus allowing a learner to choose content and tools appropriate to their differing interests, needs and skill levels;

- range and course availability can be significantly increased;

- it allows for multiple learning styles using a variety of delivery methods geared to different learners;

- it tends to be more learner-centred;

- accessibility is anytime and anywhere;

- online learning does not require physical attendance at a particular place and time;

- it can encourage greater student interaction and collaboration;

- it can encourage greater student / teacher contact;

- it enhances computer and internet skills;

- it provides global opportunities for learning.
  (www.gov.uk; www.tech-faq.com; www.kineo.com)

> **FURTHER READING**
>
> There is a considerable amount of information on the internet about study skills. You should be able to start your search using a general search engine such as Google.
>
> Both of the following books are highly recommended for anyone with a serious interest in long-term development of their learning and study skills:
>
> • Lloyd, M. & Murphy, P. (2008) *Essential Study Skills for Health and Social Care*. Exeter: Reflect Press.
>
> • Northledge, A (2007) *The Good Study Guide*. Milton Keynes: The Open University.

## Chapter summary

• The more study skills and strategies you apply and practise, the more independent and confident you can become in a learning situation.

• The style of reading should be chosen to suit the task, i.e. skimming, scanning, detailed or critical reading, and should whenever possible be as active as possible.

• To be effective, note-taking should have a purpose and be well organised.

• The basis of any essay should always begin from an understanding of what you are trying to achieve.

• The accepted basic framework for any essay is an introduction, a main text / body and a conclusion.

• Information technology and computers have a very important part to play in helping with your studies.

## References

Northledge, A. (2007) *The Good Study Guide*. Milton Keynes: The Open University.

*Oxford English Dictionary* (2012) www.oed.com (accessed 20 November 2012) www.adprima.com/studyout.htm (accessed 20 November 2012)

www.bized.co.uk/reference/studyskills/reading.htm (accessed
20 November 2012)

http://data.bolton.ac.uk/bissto/studyskills/essay/index.htm (accessed
6 January 2013)

dictionary.reference.com/browse/study?s = t&ld = 1032 (accessed
20 November 2012)

www.gre.ac.uk/studyskills/reading_skills (accessed 20 November 2012)

www.educationscotland.gov.uk/studyskills/about/index.asp (accessed
6 January 2013)

kineo.com/elearning-reports/the-benefits-of-e-learning.html (accessed
20 November 2012)

jerz.setonhill.edu/writing/academic/research/online.htm (accessed
20 November 2012)

www.litemind.com/what-is-mind-mapping (accessed 20 November 2012)

http://mail.baylorschool.org/ ~ jstover/plagiarism/notes.htm (accessed
6 January 2013)

www.mindtools.com/pages/article/newISS_01.htm (accesssed
20 November 2012)

www2.napier.ac.uk/getready/writing_presenting/essays.html (accessed
20 November 2012)

www3.northern.edu/library/faq.html (accessed 20 November 2012)

openlearn.open.ac.uk/mod/oucontent/view.php?id = 398908&direct = 1
(accessed 20 November 2012)

www.shef.ac.uk/is/current/refwrite (accessed 20 November 2012)

www.soton.ac.uk/library/resources/documents/vancouverreferencing.pdf
(accessed 20 November 2012)

www.studyskills.soton.ac.uk/studytips/reading_skills.htm (accessed
20 November 2012)

studyskills.wiki.staffs.ac.uk/Online_Resources_A_-_Z (accessed
20 November 2012)

www.tech-faq.com/e-learning.html (accessed 20 November 2012)

www.theory.org.uk/david/essaywriting.pdf (accessed 20 November 2012)

www.uefap.com/reading/readfram.htm (accessed 20 November 2012)

www.uleth.ca/lib/guides/research/display.asp?PageID = 35 (accessed 20 November 2012)

# 11
# MEDICINE, IV FLUID AND BLOOD ADMINISTRATION

As a student you will only be able to observe the administration of oral medications, intravenous (IV) fluids or blood transfusion to patients, or perhaps undertake some of these activities under direct supervision. However, it is essential that you are aware of the legislation, professional standards and local policies which govern these activities, and the aim of this chapter is to outline the considerations that are required when they are undertaken.

**Learning Outcomes**

On completion of this chapter you should be able to:

- discuss the legal and professional responsibilities of the registered nurse when administering medications, intravenous therapy and blood transfusions;
- describe the actions necessary when administering medicines, intravenous fluids and blood;
- discuss potential complications, and subsequent actions taken, in administering medicines and blood transfusions;
- use your numeracy skills to calculate accurately medicine dosages and intravenous rates.

## Introduction

Clinical placements will all have policies about medicine administration (drug rounds) and intravenous medications, and when registered you will be expected to undertake an assessment of competence (set by the employer) prior to administering any medicines. The assessment will always include an oral medicine round and, in some instances, administration of intravenous fluids and blood transfusions. Administration of intravenous drugs will be assessed separately.

A prescribed medicine is the most common treatment provided for patients in the NHS (Peate, 2006). If anything goes wrong with the administration of that medicine, the nurse is accountable in the criminal courts, the civil courts, before their employer and before the NMC (Dimond, 2011).

The NMC issues *The Code* (NMC, 2008a) as a benchmark for all nurses to adhere to when delivering care. In addition, it issues *Standards for Medicines Management* (2008b) and, while this guidance has no legal force, it establishes principles for safe practice in the management and administration of medicines by registered nurses in the UK (Dimond, 2011).

The *Standards for Medicines Management* (NMC, 2008b, p. 1) state:

> The administration of medicines is an important aspect of the professional practice of persons whose names are on the Council's register. It is not solely a mechanistic task to be performed in strict compliance with the written prescription of a medical practitioner. It requires thought and the exercise of professional judgement.....

### ACTIVITY 11.1

Take a few minutes to review *Chapter 3* on 'Legal and professional issues'. Then describe three circumstances where a registered nurse could be judged negligent in respect of administering medicines.

## Legislation concerning medicines

The key pieces of legislation that you need to be aware of are:

- Medicines Act (1968);

- Misuse of Drugs Act (1971);

- Misuse of Drugs Regulations (2001);

- Misuse of Drugs Act (Safe Custody) Regulations (1973);

- Care Standards Act (2000);

- Health Act (2006).

The *London Pharmacopoeia*, listing approved drugs, was first published in 1618 but the control of medicines in Britain can be traced back to the fifteenth century. In the nineteenth century the Pharmaceutical Society of Great Britain was formed and legislation introduced to regulate the sale of poisons. The creation of the NHS in 1948 led to the setting up of a government committee to consider the value of medicines, but it was not until 1968 that the Medicines Act introduced legislation to cover all aspects of the safety and quality of medicine management. The need for this legislation was heightened by the thalidomide tragedy in the late 1950s and early 1960s, where a medication prescribed for morning sickness caused congenital malformations when given in the first trimester of pregnancy.

Today, the current legislation controlling manufacture, supply and use of medicines is mainly found in the Medicines Act (1968), the Misuse of Drugs Act (1971) and the Misuse of Drugs Regulations (2001).

## Medicines Act (1968 and 1971) (from Dimond, 2011)

This act set up a comprehensive system of medicine controls covering:

- administrative system;

- licensing system;

- retail pharmacies;

- packing and labelling of medicinal products;

- British pharmacopoeia;

- sale and supply of medicines to the public, i.e.:

  - Prescription-only medicines (POMs) – These are medicines that may only be supplied or administered to a patient on the instruction of an appropriate practitioner (a doctor, dentist or nurse prescriber).

  - Pharmacy-only medicines – These can be purchased from a registered pharmacy, provided the sale is supervised by the pharmacist.

  - General sale list medicines (GSLs) – These do not need either a prescription or the supervision of a pharmacist and can be obtained from retail outlets.

## Misuse of Drugs Act (1971)

Controlled drugs are defined in the Misuse of Drugs Act (1971). They include those drugs which are habit-forming and certain other narcotics which have a profound effect on the central nervous system. The Act:

- lists and classifies controlled drugs;

- creates criminal offences in relation to the manufacture, supply and possession of controlled drugs;

- gives the Secretary of State power to make regulations and directions to prevent misuse of controlled drugs;

- creates advisory council on misuse of drugs;

- gives powers of search, arrest and forfeiture.

Further information can be obtained from the Medicines and Healthcare Products Regulatory Agency (MHRA) at www.mhra.gov.uk.

# Pharmacology

One of the safest, most convenient, economic and acceptable ways to administer medicines is orally, but this is not always possible as:

- the patient has to be co-operative and able to swallow the medicine;

- the chemical structures of some medicines mean that they are not absorbed (or absorbed only to a limited extent) in the small intestine; or that they can cause gross gastric and intestinal irritation; or that they are totally destroyed before they can be absorbed;

- some medicines may be absorbed by the intestine only to be inactivated by metabolism in the liver.

The rate of elimination of the medicine affects its efficiency, since the faster the body breaks down or excretes the medicine, the more rapidly the blood levels of the medicine will fall. The speed of elimination is the main factor in determining the duration of action of a medicine. Medicines are eliminated by:

- breaking down or combining with a chemical so that they are no longer pharmacologically active – usually by enzymes in the liver;

- being excreted by the kidney, but if kidney disease is present this may be delayed and the medicine accumulates in the blood stream (e.g. antibiotics);

- in a few cases, excretion through the lungs (e.g. anaesthetic agents).

# Administration of medicines

While you are practising there are many aspects of medicine administration that you, as a registered nurse, need to be aware of. Dimond (2011) suggests that the main areas of concern are those shown in *Figure 11.1*. Some of these headings are explored more fully in the next few pages; others may be found in *Standards for Medicines Management* (NMC, 2008b).

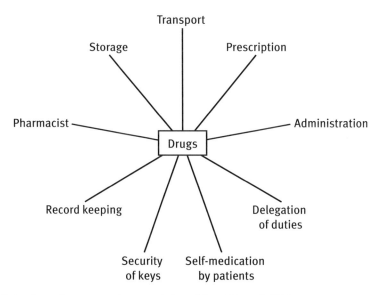

*Figure 11.1 – Areas that concern the nurse (adapted from Dimond, 2011)*

## Prescription

There are several ways that medicines are prescribed. Generally a doctor, dentist or nurse prescriber is responsible for patient diagnosis and initiation of medicine treatment.

The prescription they write must include:

- the patient's full name, date of birth, weight and allergies;

- the generic (proper) name of the medicine (not the trade name), strength, dose, form (elixir, tabs, etc.), route of administration and frequency to be taken;

- a signature and date by the doctor / nurse prescriber.

The prescription must be indelible and legible. It should also state the duration of the course of medication before a patient review should take place.

### Nurse prescribing

Primary legislation permitting nurse prescribing is set out in the Medicinal Products: Prescription by Nurses Act (1992) and subsequent amendments. This allows nurses and midwives who have undertaken further training and recorded their qualification with the NMC to become nurse or midwife prescribers. There are two levels of prescribers – community practitioner nurse prescribers, and independent and supplementary nurse and midwife prescribers.

### FURTHER INFORMATION

If you wish to know more about nurse prescribing, access the NMC website at www.nmc-uk.org and read their position statement, or see pages 23–24 of *Standards for Medicines Management* (NMC, 2008b).

### Remote prescription or direction to administer (NMC, 2008b, Standard 11)

Instruction by telephone to administer a previously unprescribed medicine is not acceptable. In exceptional circumstances, where a medication (not including controlled drugs) has been previously prescribed and the prescriber is unable to issue a new prescription, but where changes in the dose are considered necessary, the use of IT (email, text message or fax) is the preferred method. This must be followed up by a new prescription confirming the changes within a given time period (usually 24 hours).

Each hospital / care home will have a policy about taking telephone orders, and it will be your responsibility when a registered nurse to become familiar with them in your clinical area.

### Patient group direction (PGD)

A PGD is a written instruction for the supply and/or administration of medicines to certain groups of patients that fit certain criteria within the directions, without the need for a prescription or an instruction from a prescriber. PGDs are drawn up locally by doctors (or dentists, pharmacists and other health care professionals), and **must** be signed by either a doctor or dentist **and** a pharmacist. A PGD is not a form of prescribing, and unlike prescribing, health care professionals entitled to work with a PGD do not require any additional formal qualification. However, employers have a responsibility to ensure that only fully competent, trained health care professionals use PGDs, and may specify local training and assessment of competence. Students cannot supply or administer medicines under a PGD; however, you are expected to understand the principles and be involved in the process (NMC, 2008b, p. 18).

PGDs cannot be delegated and the same nurse or health care practitioner must both supply and administer the medicine. They are not appropriate where a range of different medicines need to be administered at the same time.

> **FURTHER INFORMATION**
>
> For further information about PGDs visit www.dh.gov.uk and type 'HSC 2000/026: Patient group directions' into the search engine.

## The pharmacist

In the UK, the pharmacist is legally responsible for the supply and distribution of drugs in accordance with the law. However, in some cases, nurses who have had additional training may dispense medicines, if this is in line with the hospital policy where they work *and* with the written instructions of a medical practitioner. The role of a pharmacist also includes that of being a resource person for medicine information, and they are responsible for checking that any newly prescribed medicine will not interact dangerously with, or nullify, any existing medication.

All medicines must be clearly and concisely labelled and should describe the contents, including:

- the patient's name;

- the name of the drug;

- the strength;

- the dose;

- the frequency;

- the directions for use;

- any special instructions (such as storage, precautions, etc.);

- the dispensing date (and expiry date if appropriate);

- the name and address of the person who sells or supplies the medicinal product;

- the words "Keep out of the reach of children" or words of direction bearing a similar meaning (for example, "Keep out of the reach and sight of children").

(NMC, 2008b, p. 82)

If the label appears to have been tampered with or altered in any way it must be reported and returned to the pharmacy immediately.

The responsibility for storing medications also lies with the pharmacist, in conjunction with the senior nurse (ward manager) in a hospital setting, or with the manager and senior nurse in a private institution. Responsibility for the administration of medicines lies with individual registered nurses (or the manager in a residential home). All medicines must be kept in locked cupboards. Individual medicines and some stock items can be held in a mobile medicine trolley and when this trolley is not in use it must be secured to a wall by a locking device, or kept in a locked cupboard.

## ACTIVITY 11.2

Look up three drugs you have seen administered in your clinical area. What are the potential side-effects / contra-indications of these medications? Are there any drugs they are incompatible with? You might like to register at the website of eBNF which can be found at www.bnf.org (you need to register, but it's free) or use www.medicines.org.uk/emc.

## The nurse's role in the administration of medicines

Students must never administer or supply medicinal products without direct supervision (NMC, 2008b, Standard 18). Registered nurses who have undergone an assessment for administering medicines must only administer medicines according to the patient's individual needs and in accordance with national, professional and local policies.

For any medicine being administered in a health care setting there are some details which must be on the patient's medicines administration chart (MAR). The MAR must be clearly and indelibly written or computer generated and it must contain:

- patient's name and date of birth;
- weight, if dosage of medication is related to patient's weight;
- medication prescribed by the proper (not generic) name;
- strength of drug;
- dose of medication;
- frequency of administration;
- route of administration;
- start and finish dates.

It must also be signed and dated by the authorised prescriber.

Before administering any medicine (NMC, 2008b, Standard 8) the registered nurse must:

- be certain of the identity of the patient to whom the medicine is to be administered;
- check that the patient is not allergic to the medicine before administering it;
- know the therapeutic uses of the medicine to be administered, its normal dosage, side-effects, precautions and contra-indications;
- be aware of the patient's plan of care (care plan or pathway);
- check that the prescription or the label on the medicine dispensed is clearly written and unambiguous;

- check the expiry date (where it exists) of the medicine to be administered;

- have considered the dosage, weight where appropriate, method of administration, route and timing. This is often referred to as the 'five rights':

  - right drug

  - right dose

  - right route

  - right time

  - right patient

Furthermore, when administering any medication the registered nurse must:

- administer or withhold in the context of the patient's condition (for example, digoxin is not usually to be given if the pulse is below 60) and co-existing therapies, for example, physiotherapy;

- contact the prescriber or another authorised prescriber without delay where contra-indications to the prescribed medicine are discovered, where the patient develops a reaction to the medicine, or where assessment of the patient indicates that the medicine is no longer suitable (see Standard 25);

- make a clear, accurate and immediate record of all medicine administered, intentionally withheld or refused by the patient, ensuring the signature is clear and legible; it is also your responsibility to ensure that a record is made when delegating the task of administering medicine.

In addition:

- where medication is not given, the reason for not doing so must be recorded;

- any prescription-only medicine, general sales list or pharmacy medication may be administered with a single signature;

- substances for injection must not be prepared in advance of their immediate use and medicines must not be administered if they have been drawn into a syringe by another practitioner when not in the presence of the practitioner administering them (NMC, 2008b, Standard 14).

### Covert administration of medicines

Disguising medication in the absence of informed consent of the patient may be regarded as deception, and anyone undertaking this practice must be convinced that they are doing this 'in the patient's best interests' and be aware that they are accountable for this action. The NMC (2007) states that covert medicine administration should only be performed in life-saving circumstances or to prevent deterioration of a patient's condition, or to ensure improvement of a patient's physical or mental health.

Registered nurses must be assured that they have the support (or otherwise) of the rest of the multiprofessional team for covertly administering medicines, and this should be recorded. Each organisation involved in health care should have a policy or protocol on the covert administration of medicines and you should be familiar with the one in your clinical area.

### Crushing medication

Many patients are unable to swallow tablets or capsules whole, and the crushing or opening of capsules is often a method used to administer medication to such patients. However, in doing this you may alter the chemical properties of the medication, and also contravene legal issues surrounding the crushing of tablets (NMC, 2007):

- the crushing of tablets, in most cases, renders them 'unlicensed' – consequently the manufacturer may assume no liability for any harm that may ensue to the patient or the person administering it;

- under the Medicines Act (1968), only medical and dental practitioners can authorise the administration of 'unlicensed' medicines; it is therefore illegal to crush a tablet before administration without the authorisation of the prescriber;

- when an 'unlicensed' medicine is authorised to be administered, a percentage of the liability for any harm that might ensue will lie with the administering nurse.

Therefore if the patient is unable to swallow tablets, an alternative such as a liquid should be prescribed instead. If there is no alternative preparation of the medication, then crushing should take place only following consultation with the prescriber and pharmacist, and this must be recorded.

## Recording of medicine administration

The NMC (2008b, Standard 8) states with regard to recording medicine administration:

> You must make a clear, accurate and immediate record of all medicine administered, intentionally withheld or refused by the patient, ensuring the signature is clear and legible; it is also your responsibility to ensure that a record is made when delegating the task of administering medicine.

In addition, where medication is not given, the reason for not doing so must be recorded.

## Controlled drugs

Controlled drugs are defined in The Misuse of Drugs Act (1971). They include those drugs which are habit-forming and certain other narcotics that have a profound effect on the central nervous system.

### Custody of controlled drugs

Controlled drugs must be kept in a locked safe or receptacle within a locked cupboard with a warning light to show when the cupboard is open. The policy for safe custody and administration of controlled drugs must be clearly laid down in local policies which all nurses are responsible for reading and understanding.

### Administration of controlled drugs (NMC, 2008b, Standard 8)

Controlled drugs must be administered in line with relevant legislation and local policies. Students can be a second signatory, as long as they have witnessed the whole administration process.

---

**FURTHER INFORMATION**

For further information visit www.dh.gov.uk and search for 'Safer management of controlled drugs: Guidance on standard operating procedures'.

---

## Self-administration

Some clinical areas have adopted a local policy for self-administration of medicines. As with all policies, you need to become familiar with their content before taking part in this procedure.

The registered nurse has a responsibility for the initial and continued assessment of patients who are self-administering their medications (NMC, 2008b, Standard 9). They also need to be assured that these patients are aware of the medicines they are taking and why, the correct dosages and possible side-effects to look for.

## Disposal of medicines

In NHS establishments all medicines that are no longer required or are out of date must be returned to the pharmacy. In care homes disposal of unwanted medication is via a clinical waste company. In any establishment only single doses of medicines that are not administered for any reason may be disposed of down a sluice or toilet system.

A single dose of a controlled drug which requires destruction may be disposed of in a sluice or toilet system, but two people, one of whom must be a registered nurse, must witness the disposal and enter the fact in the Controlled Drug Register.

> **FURTHER INFORMATION**
>
> Further information about medicine administration can be found on the NMC website (www.nmc-uk.org) – search for 'medicines management'.

# Principles of practice

While no one intends to make a mistake when administering medicines, unfortunately they do happen. However, by following correct procedures the opportunity for mistakes can be reduced, and the following pages explore what an error is, and how best practice can be promoted.

A medication error can be made by:

- doctors;
- pharmacists;
- nurses;
- health care assistants;
- any other health care professional involved with medication.

A medication error occurs when one or more of the following occurs:

- the wrong medication is administered;
- the wrong patient is administered the medication;
- the patient receives an over- or underdose;
- a dose is missed or late;
- the medication chart is not signed;
- the medication is changed from its licensed formulation (e.g. dissolved in tea).

It has been stated that over 90% of errors may not be reported (Meikle, 2000). There are many reasons for this but perhaps the key two are not realising an error has been made and fear of the outcome if an error is declared.

An open culture is advocated as the best approach when managing any error in the work place (NMC, 2008b, p. 60). This is encouraged to ensure prompt reporting for the wellbeing of both patient and staff, and ensuring that learning takes place from the error made, so that it does not happen again. Therefore, all errors and incidents must be investigated, taking in a full account of the context and circumstances.

## Preventing errors

In some instances there may be an argument that it is the working environment, rather than the individual nurse responsible for administering medicines, that causes the incidence of error to increase. A common example of this is being interrupted during the medicine round. By using the approach that it is a team concern, it may be easier to explore how errors can be prevented. In this way the culture of the workplace can move from one that manages mistakes to one that proactively works to eliminate or minimise the risk of error.

Principles of best practice can be identified as points of safety. That is, if all possibilities are considered, the risk can be significantly reduced or eliminated.

These can be listed under three headings:

### Knowledge

- Be aware of correct storage, expiration dates, labelling, etc;
- Know therapeutic dosages, side-effects, contra-indications, precautions;
- Be aware of where to obtain information;
- Consider dosage, timing and route in context with patient history.

### Communication

- Ensure clear record keeping;
- Ensure appropriate and clearly written prescriptions;
- Ensure allergies are clearly written and the appropriate people are informed;
- Ensure patient consent and understanding, whenever possible;
- Be aware of the patient's care plan.

### Procedure

- Ensure clear procedures that are understood by all staff;
- Confirm patient identity;
- Ensure policies for medication management are known to all and regularly reviewed;
- Ensure that patients are regularly reviewed and relevant personnel notified when a reaction is noted or treatment no longer appears effective.

## Adverse reactions

There are a number of ways patients can react to medicines, and as a student you need to be aware of them.

**Overdose** gives an increased pharmacological effect.

**Intolerance** or excess effect of a normal dose – the medicine is not metabolised or excreted by the liver or the kidney, and therefore stays in the body longer than anticipated.

**Side-effects** unrelated to the primary purpose for which the medicine is given. They are *not* inevitable, in that other medicines with the same primary action might not produce them (e.g. some antihistamines cause drowsiness, others do not; some analgesics cause respiratory depression, others do not).

**Secondary side-effects** result from the normal action of the medicine, but the medicine may develop more than one action (e.g. antibiotics cause diarrhoea because they are incompletely absorbed from the small intestine and therefore kill off some of the bacteria the body relies on for normal function when they reach the large intestine).

**Hypersensitivity** is a reaction caused when the patient has been exposed to the medicine on a previous occasion. The exposure has resulted in the production of an antibody against the medicine. Antibodies are proteins formed in the body as a result of the introduction of a foreign substance (an antigen), which then become attached to the surface of certain cells which are scattered around the body. In an allergic (anaphylactic) reaction a second dose of the medicine is given, and the antigen (medicine) combines with the antibody, causing histamine to be released which causes an acute **anaphylactic reaction**.

## Anaphylaxis

The following outlines the features of an anaphylactic reaction and the Resuscitation Council's guidelines (2010) for treatment of anaphylaxis. Anaphylactic reactions vary in severity and progress may be rapid or slow, and in rare cases manifestations may be delayed by a few hours or persist for more than 24 hours.

Anaphylaxis is likely when all of the following three criteria are met:

• sudden onset and rapid progression of symptoms;

• life-threatening airway and/or breathing and/or circulation problems;

• skin and/or mucosal changes (flushing, urticaria, angioedema).

Exposure to a known allergen for the patient supports the diagnosis, but:

• skin or mucosal changes alone are not a sign of an anaphylactic reaction;

- skin and mucosal changes can be subtle or absent in up to twenty per cent of reactions (some patients may only have a decrease in blood pressure, i.e. a circulation problem);

- there can also be gastrointestinal symptoms (e.g. vomiting, abdominal pain, incontinence).

(Resuscitation Council, 2010)

### Treatment for anaphylaxis

Stop trigger (i.e. drug administration)

Rapid assessment:

**A**irway: look for and relieve airway obstruction; call for help early if there are signs of obstruction.

**B**reathing: look for and treat bronchospasm and signs of respiratory distress.

**C**irculation: colour, pulse and BP.

**D**isability: assess whether responding or unconscious.

**E**xposure: assess skin with adequate exposure, but avoid excess heat loss.

Consider anaphylaxis when there is compatible history of rapid-onset severe allergic-type reaction with respiratory difficulty and/or hypotension, especially if there are skin changes present.

**Give high-flow oxygen**: Use a mask with an oxygen reservoir (greater than 10 litres per minute to prevent reservoir collapse).

**Lay the patient flat**: Raise the legs (this must be done with care, as it may worsen any breathing problems).

**Administer adrenaline (epinephrine)**: Adrenaline causes the blood vessels to constrict (become narrower), which raises blood pressure and reduces swelling. It also causes the airways to open, relieving breathing difficulties, and suppresses the release of histamine.

Doses: intramuscularly (IM) in the anterolateral aspect of the middle third of the thigh (safe, easy, effective):

Adult IM dose 0.5 mg IM ( = 500 micrograms = 0.5 mL of 1:1000) adrenaline

Child IM dose (the equivalent volume of 1:1000 adrenaline (epinephrine) is shown in brackets)

> 12 years: 500 micrograms IM (0.5 mL), i.e. the same as the adult dose. 300 micrograms (0.3 mL) if the child is small or prepubertal. Between 6 and 12 years: 300 micrograms IM (0.3 mL).

< 6 years: 150 micrograms IM (0.15 mL).

IM adrenaline (epinephrine) should be repeated after 5 minutes if there is no clinical improvement. Patients requiring repeated IM doses may benefit from IV adrenaline (epinephrine). In these circumstances, expert help is required as soon as possible.

**Airway**: Establish airway (in anaphylaxis, airway obstruction from tissue swelling is difficult to overcome and early expert intubation is often needed).

**IV fluid challenge**: Insert one or more large-bore IV cannulae (enable the highest flow). Use intraosseous access in children when IV access is difficult.

Give a rapid fluid challenge:

Adults – 500 mL of warmed crystalloid solution (e.g. Hartmann's or 0.9% saline) in 5–10 minutes if the patient is normotensive or 1 L if the patient is hypotensive.

Children – give 20 mL/kg of warmed crystalloid.

**Drugs**: Chlorphenamine

      Hydrocortisone

Continuing respiratory deterioration requires further treatment with a bronchodilator, such as salbutamol (inhaled or IV), ipratropium (inhaled), aminophylline (IV) or magnesium sulphate (IV – unlicensed indication). Magnesium is a vasodilator and can compound hypotension and shock. For doses, refer to the *British National Formulary* (BNF).

Monitor: Pulse, blood pressure, ECG.

(Resuscitation Council, 2010)

**It is very important that you know where the resuscitation equipment is kept in your clinical area and familiarise yourself with its contents.**

## ACTIVITY 11.3

Read the following article and then identify and comment on the clauses of *The Code: Standards of Conduct, Performance and Ethics for Nurses and Midwives* (NMC, 2008a) and *Standards for Medicines Management* (NMC, 2008b) which David breached.

*(Reproduced with permission from the British Journal of Nursing)*

### Staff nurse removed from nursing register for mis-management of drug rounds

*British Journal of Nursing* (2005) **14(18)**: 953: Professional Misconduct Series.

David was a staff nurse employed by a large hospital trust in the north of England. He usually worked night duty and was known for his efficiency in completing nursing tasks.

The ward David worked on contained many older patients, who were recovering from various medical interventions. Debra, who was a new staff nurse, came to work opposite shifts with David and could not believe how quickly he completed his drug rounds. One day she thought she discovered the reason why this was so: she found out that one of David's patients had been signed off as receiving his drugs when in fact he had not received them.

This came to light over a weekend when it was difficult to obtain certain drugs as the pharmacy was closed. Debra remembered giving the last dose of a drug to a patient and then putting the empty container on the pharmacy trolley. When she followed on from David again she was surprised to note that David had signed off as having given the drug which she had previously sent back empty to the pharmacy. At first Debra thought David may have found another stock of the drug, but when she checked again this appeared to be untrue.

When she challenged David about the incident he shrugged it off by saying that he had signed the prescription chart before he had checked the stock. He apologised for the oversight and gave an assurance that there would be no further errors on his part.

Debra accepted David's explanation and decided not to take any further action. Unfortunately when Debra carried out a drug round a few days later she found two pots in the medicine trolley, both of which contained supposedly dispensed medication. One pot contained dispensed temazepam syrup, which she identified because of the distinctive smell, and the other pot contained two tablets of MST 10mg, which she recognised from the size and colour.

## ACTIVITY 11.3 continued

When asked why he had not administered the MST, David replied that he had no idea, adding that he might have been called away and had then forgotten. David also said that he left the temazepam in the trolley to remind him that he had not administered it. Debra mentioned this to the senior nurse, who arranged for David to undertake a training session regarding the procedures for the administration of medicines.

When Debra came to undertake a monthly drug count and audit of medicines she found that there were unexplained surpluses of medication, particularly for the patients who were more confused. Debra wrote in her statement that she had returned the surplus stock to the pharmacy during the previous month and was surprised, therefore, that the discrepancies were so large.

Shortly after this incident, when David was on duty another discrepancy occurred. This involved large quantities of medication being checked and found exactly as they were the previous evening. A seal on a new bottle of Alupent was intact despite it being prescribed for a patient. David claimed that the reason for the same levels was that he borrowed medication for other patients. Unfortunately he was unable to identify whose medication he had borrowed and could not remember why it had been necessary for him to borrow another patient's medication when that patient's medication was also in the drug trolley.

When asked about the other patients who had been signed off as receiving their medications yet the stock levels were the same, he replied that he did not know why he had not administered the medication.

David's case was referred to the NMC, where he reiterated that he could not explain why he did not give the patients their medications. One possible excuse was that he had been suffering from stress since his divorce. David was not referred to the health committee but admitted that he could not give a reasonable explanation for his actions. He was charged on 10 counts of making errors in the administration of drugs and his name was removed from the register for a minimum of five years.

Note: this case is in a series based on actual true cases which were reported to the NMC. Compiled by George Castledine, Professor and Consultant of General Nursing, University of Central England, Birmingham, and Dudley Group of Hospitals NHS Trust.

# Intravenous (IV) therapy

Health care employers will assess registered nurses prior to allowing them to administer intravenous fluids. As a student you may undertake this procedure under direct supervision.

Nurses play a crucial role in the management of IV therapy and the prevention or early detection of complications (Dougherty and Lamb, 2008). Depending on the solutions used, and the condition of the patient, IV therapy may be continuous, intermittent or given as a single dose injection. It can be administered either via a peripheral cannula or central catheter; however, peripheral venous cannulation is the commonest method used for intravenous therapy (Waitt et al., 2004).

## Indications for peripheral venous cannulation

These are:

- intravenous fluids;

- limited parenteral nutrition;

- blood and blood products;

- drug administration (continuous or intermittent);

- prophylactic use before procedures;

- prophylactic use in unstable patients.

## Contra-indications and cautions for peripheral venous cannulation

These are:

- inflammation or infection of the insertion site;

- forearm veins in patients with renal failure (may be needed for arteriovenous fistulae);

- irritant drugs into small veins with low flow rates (i.e. leg and foot veins).

## Crystalloids and colloids

There are two types of fluids that are used for intravenous infusions: crystalloids and colloids. Crystalloids are aqueous solutions of mineral salts or other water-soluble molecules, whereas colloids contain larger insoluble molecules, such as gelatin. Blood itself is a colloid. The most commonly used crystalloid fluid is normal saline, a solution of sodium chloride at 0.9% concentration, which is close to the concentration in the blood. Ringer's lactate is another isotonic solution often used for large-volume fluid replacement. A solution of 5% dextrose in water is often used if the patient is at risk of having low blood sugar or high sodium. The choice of fluids may also depend on the chemical properties of any medications being given.

## Intravenous devices

Prior to the commencement of intravenous therapy certain factors must be taken into account:

• the length of time for which the pathway is needed;

• the suitability of the patient's veins;

• the nature of the intended procedure;

• type of devices used to administer the therapy.

The flow of any infusion fluid may be influenced by:

• the height of the infusion bag – the chamber should be no more than 1m from the cannula;

• solution being infused – the more viscous the solution, the slower it will flow;

• temperature of the fluid;

• physical condition of the patient:

  • vein spasm / obstructed vein

  • changes in blood pressure

  • patient movement

  • restricted clothing and equipment (e.g. blood pressure cuff)

• size of the cannula – the larger the lumen, the faster the flow:

  • for infusions of viscous fluid (e.g. blood) and rapid infusions, 14–16 gauge cannula should be used

- for crystalloid infusions, 18–20 gauge cannula should be used

- for intermittent administration of drugs, 20–24 gauge cannula should be used

The choices of cannulae are:

- winged infusion set (butterfly) for single drug dose only;

- short catheter for infusions of short duration;

- central catheter for long-term therapy.

Peripheral cannulae should be changed routinely after 48–72 hours (Waitt *et al.*, 2004) because the rate of phlebitis increases with time.

---

**ACTIVITY 11.4**

What type of solutions would you administer via the following?

a. Winged infusion set

b. Short cannula

c. Central catheter

---

## Choice of vein

Veins on the non-dominant forearm are most suitable, especially if the cannula has to remain in position for any length of time. Veins on the dorsum of the hand are easiest to cannulate, but are more uncomfortable for the patient and more liable to block. Veins in the lower limb should be avoided where possible because of the increased incidence of thrombophlebitis and thrombosis (Waitt *et al.*, 2004).

## Choice of administration (giving) set

- Blood set – for blood and blood products with integral filter.

- Solution set – standard administration set for most fluids.

- Burette set – for more accurate fluid delivery and in children.

## Managing the infusion site

### Observation of the site

The cannula site should be inspected at least once a day and every time IV drugs are administered. Observe for redness (phlebitis, thrombophlebitis), heat (infection) and swelling (extravasation or infiltration). The insertion site should not be painful.

### Types of dressing

The peripheral IV site should be covered with a dressing that is sterile, easy to apply and remove, keeps the site free from exogenous infection, secures the cannula in place and allows easy visual inspection of the site. It should only be changed if the dressing becomes wet or bloodstained or haemoserous fluid collects around the site (Dougherty and Lamb, 2008).

### Prevention of contamination

Asepsis is the key preventative measure in reducing the likelihood of infection, and hand washing is the most important aspect of this. Prior to any manipulation of the cannula, IV fluid, administration set or IV site, or change of dressing, thorough hand washing must take place, and in most instances sterile gloves must be worn (check your local policy). Minimal handling of the administration system will also help prevent infection (Dougherty and Lamb, 2008).

## Methicillin-resistant *Staphylococcus aureus* (MRSA)

MRSA (methicillin-resistant *Staphylococcus aureus*) is a strain of *Staphylococcus aureus* which is resistant to methicillin and other antibiotics, and this resistance has been evident for the last 40 years (RCN, 2005). It colonises the skin, particularly the nose, skin folds, hairline, perineum and navel and commonly survives in these areas without causing infection. The patient only becomes clinically infected if the organism invades the skin or deeper tissues and multiplies. Transmission is by person-to-person contact or via equipment, and MRSA has been found to be prevalent in patients with intravenous devices. The symptoms are the same as for any infection, and include redness, swelling and tenderness at the site of infection.

In order to reduce the spread of MRSA, nurses should ensure:

- hand washing before and after contact with every patient or potentially contaminated equipment;

- hand washing after removal of gloves;

- keeping the environment as clean and dry as possible;

- thorough cleaning and drying of all equipment after use.

(RCN, 2005)

> **FURTHER INFORMATION**
>
> Further information about infection control in general can be found on the RCN website (www.rcn.org.uk). The document *Wipe it Out: Essential Practice for Infection Prevention and Control* is very helpful.

## Comfort

The psychological as well as the physical comfort of the patient must be considered. If high standards are maintained throughout the procedure then physical safety will be met. Giving the patient adequate explanation and information about the procedure in terms that they understand will help to meet their psychological needs.

## Intravenous fluids

All fluid to be infused should be checked and inspected prior to use in order to prevent contamination / infection, and if there is any doubt the fluid should be returned to the pharmacy. Also:

- check the packaging is intact;

- inspect the container for punctures, air bubbles, discoloration, haziness and particles;

- check the expiry date of the fluid;

- record the batch number.

## Infusion devices / pumps

An infusion pump infuses fluids, medication or nutrients into a patient's circulatory system. It is generally used intravenously, although subcutaneous, arterial and epidural infusions are used. They are designed to deliver measured amounts of drug or fluid over a period of time to achieve a desired therapeutic response.

### Volumetric pumps

Volumetric pumps are used when a large volume of fluid needs to be administered (e.g. parenteral nutrition). They work by calculating the volume delivered with the rate selected in millilitres per hour, and are capable of accurate delivery over a wide range of flow rates.

### Syringe pumps

These are low-volume, high-accuracy devices designed to infuse at low flow rates where the rate is controlled by the drive speed of the piston attached to the syringe plunger. They are useful where small volumes of concentrated drugs need to be infused.

### Patient Controlled Analgesia (PCA) pumps

These are syringe pumps, but their distinguishing feature is that they can deliver doses on demand, when the patient pushes a button. Doses can be limited by a designated maximum amount. This method of delivering analgesia increases patient satisfaction as less sedation is required.

## Complications of intravenous therapy

### Infection

Infections can result from intrinsically contaminated equipment or fluids, but the vast majority are due to extrinsic contamination. Dougherty and Lister (2011) maintain that good hand washing is the fundamental technique in greatly reducing the normal skin flora that is capable of causing sepsis. Minimal handling of any part of the IV delivery system and maintaining a 'closed system' with as few connections as possible will also help prevent infection.

For optimal skin preparation, injection sites on administration sets or injection caps should be cleaned using an alcohol-based antiseptic for a minimum of 30 seconds and allowed time to air dry (Pratt *et al.*, 2007). Administration sets should be changed according to their use, type of device and type of solution, and the set must be labelled with the date and time of change (RCN, 2005; NPSA, 2007). This is usually between 48 and 72 hours. Infusion bags should not be left hanging for more than 24 hours.

The insertion site must be checked (at least) once daily (RCN, 2005) or whenever the closed system is broken (e.g. when administering drugs, changing administration sets, etc.). Many hospitals have a check list for this included with the patient's care plan.

To treat an infection, stop the infusion and remove the cannula. Follow hospital policy about sending the catheter tip for bacterial analysis.

### Infiltration / extravasation

This is caused when the cannula slips out of the vein wall and the infused fluid accumulates in the surrounding tissues. To treat, stop the infusion and remove the cannula.

### Phlebitis

Phlebitis is an inflammation of a vein and is caused most frequently by irritation of the vein wall. To treat, the infusion should be stopped and the cannula removed.

### Thrombophlebitis

This is the inflammation of a vein associated with thrombus formation. To treat, stop the infusion and remove the cannula.

### Precipitation

Precipitation is the incompatibility between two fluids (e.g. blood and glucose). Stop the infusion and remove the cannula. Change both the giving set and the solution.

### Air embolus

This is not a common problem, but nevertheless can be fatal, particularly in central lines. Air enters the venous circulation via an intravenous line and can block blood flow. The amount of air required to cause fatalities is uncertain. The treatment is to turn the patient onto their left side and lower the head of the bed to prevent air entering pulmonary artery. In addition, oxygen should be administered.

### Circulation overload

This occurs when an infusion is given too quickly and causes the patient to exhibit tachycardia, distended neck veins, dyspnoea and respiratory distress. Treatment is symptomatic, along with restriction of fluids and possible use of diuretics.

### Speed shock

This happens when certain drugs or chemical-rich fluids are infused too rapidly. It causes toxic concentrations to accumulate within the circulation and produces shock-like symptoms such as tachycardia, hypotension, progressive syncope and collapse. The treatment is to stop the infusion and treat the symptoms.

# Blood transfusion

A blood transfusion is defined as the administration of whole blood or any of its components into the bloodstream to correct or treat a clinical abnormality (Anderson *et al.*, 2001). The first blood transfusion is reported to have been in 1492 when Pope Innocent was given the blood of three Roman citizens – unfortunately all of them died. In the centuries that followed the technique developed, the key milestone being in 1901 when Karl Landsteiner discovered that not all blood was the same and developed the ABO blood grouping that is universally used today. The Rhesus system was discovered in 1940.

## Blood groups

The ABO system classifies human red blood cells into 4 main groups: A, B, AB and O. The blood group of a person is determined by the absence or presence of A and B antigens on their red blood cells.

**Antigen:** A substance which the body regards as foreign or potentially dangerous, which adheres to the surface of existing red cells, and against which the body produces an antibody.

**Antibody:** A protein which is formed in the body in response to an antigen and circulates within the plasma in an effort to render the antigen harmless. The body inherits established major antibodies, such as in the ABO and Rhesus blood grouping systems.

## The Rhesus system

Approximately 85% of the western population also have D antigen on their red blood cells, which is termed Rhesus positive. Those who are termed Rhesus negative have no D antigen and therefore no naturally-occurring antibodies. The antibody could, however, be produced by the body in response to exposure to D antigen, for example following transfusion of

Rh D+ blood, or during pregnancy if the father is Rh D+ and the mother Rh D– (Dougherty and Lister, 2011).

**Table 11.1** The compatibility for blood transfusion between people with the various blood groups. People with AB blood can receive blood from any group, and those with O blood are universal donors.

| Group | Antigens | Antibodies | Compatible donor for | Compatible recipient of |
|-------|----------|------------|----------------------|-------------------------|
| A | A | Anti B | A, AB | A, O |
| B | B | Anti A | B, AB | B, O |
| AB | A + B | None | AB | A, B, AB, O |
| O | None | Anti A + Anti B | A, B, AB, O | O |

## Indications for blood transfusion

Indications for blood transfusions are:

- to replace any blood loss during surgery, or as a result of haemorrhage;

- to replace a deficiency of a blood product (e.g. platelets);

- to increase the oxygen-carrying component, as in anaemia;

- to increase the circulating blood volume, as in hypovolaemic shock.

(Dougherty and Lister, 2011)

## Managing the transfusion

The transfusion of blood and its components is usually safe and uneventful; however, there are associated risks which have been highlighted in recent years. In 2005 the Blood Safety and Quality Regulations (2005) came into effect, which cover the collection, testing, processing, storage and distribution of blood and blood components.

There are many blood products currently available, all of which have varying shelf lives, storage and transfusion requirements. However, certain key observations have to be made for patients receiving blood products:

- all patients must have an identity wristband with their name, date of birth and unique hospital number clearly written or printed;

- all patients should be advised of possible adverse effects and asked to report them immediately: anxiousness, fever, rigors, flushing, rash, loin pain, backache, transfusion site pain, shortness of breath;

- patients should be in a highly visible area in the ward;

- initial recordings of pulse and temperature;

- further check of pulse and temperature at 15 minutes once unit commenced – adverse reactions often occur within the first 15 minutes of transfusion (Gray and Illingworth, 2006);

- hourly checks of pulse and temperature thereafter;

- unit of blood component must be completed within 4 hours – over 4 hours increases risk of reaction and complications;

- administration sets should be changed every 12 hours or after administration of every second unit;

- monitor fluid balance;

- maintain clinical records of whole procedure including blood component labels;

- keep all empty blood component bags until transfusion is completed.

(Dougherty and Lister, 2011)

### *Filters*

Blood must be administered through a blood administration set as it has an integral filter to remove red cell debris, leucocytes, platelets and fibrin strands that clump together. There should be no need to use additional filters unless the patient is receiving multiple units or cardiac bypass surgery.

### *Checks for blood product to be transfused*

- Expiry date;

- Visual inspection of blood component for signs of clumping, discoloration, damage or leaks;

- Positive identification of patient. Check patient details against wrist band and details on blood product;

- Check that information on compatibility label matches details on blood component (blood group, donation label).

## Transfusion reactions

The transfusion of any blood product carries with it the potential of a transfusion reaction which could be immediate or delayed.

### *Acute haemolytic reaction*

This is directly related to incompatibilities in the ABO blood group system, for example when blood containing anti-A antibodies (group B) mixes with blood containing A antigens (group A), the donor antibodies attach to the surface of the recipient's red blood cells, causing cells to clump together. Eventually these clumped cells can plug small blood vessels, leading to disseminated intravascular coagulation.

This antibody / antigen reaction activates a process that promotes and accelerates red blood cell destruction, which in turn causes free haemoglobin to be released into the blood stream. This damages the kidney tubules and can lead to renal failure and death.

Reactions can occur after as little as 5 mL of blood being transfused, and are almost wholly preventable, since reactions result from incorrect blood cross-matching, clerical error or checking errors at the bedside (Dougherty and Lister, 2011).

*Features* of an acute haemolytic reaction include: hypotension, pyrexia, chills, agitation, pain at the cannula site, lumbar pain, facial flushing, bleeding from wound sites and chest pain.

*Action:* stop infusion immediately. Treat hypotension and give appropriate therapy for disseminated intravascular coagulation.

### *Anaphylactic reactions*

These are rare and usually due to production of antibodies by patients who have had a previous blood transfusion. The antibodies in plasma combine with antigens in donated red blood cells, causing histamine to be released, which in turn causes an acute anaphylactic reaction. The risk of this can be lessened by transfusing packed cells where 80% of the plasma (where the antibodies circulate) has been removed.

*Features* of anaphylaxis include: angio-oedema, urticaria, dyspnoea, hypotension, acute irreversible asthma or laryngeal oedema, rhinitis, conjunctivitis, abdominal pain, vomiting, diarrhoea, sense of impending doom, skin colour (either flushed or pale) and cardiovascular collapse.

*Action*: stop infusion and resuscitate patient.

### Pyogenic reaction

This is probably the most common cause of fever and not considered serious. Pyogens are the breakdown material from bacteria in blood before sterilisation.

*Features* include pyrexia, but without signs of shock, followed by the pyrexia subsiding if the transfusion is slowed.

*Table 11.2* outlines the different characteristics of a haemolytic reaction and an anaphylactic reaction.

**Table 11.2** The differences between haemolytic and anaphylactic reactions.

| Haemolytic | Anaphylactic |
|---|---|
| Facial flushing | Shock |
| Chills | Abdominal cramps |
| Backache / loin pain | Respiratory distress |
| Rigors | Rash |
| Chest pain | Facial oedema |
| Hypotension | Bronchial spasm |
| Oliguria | |
| **Renal failure and shock Treatment** | **Anaphylactic shock Treatment** |
| Oxygen | Adrenaline |
| IV fluids | Antihistamine |
| Diuretics | Hydrocortisone |
| Adrenaline (if indicated) | Diuretics (if indicated) |

# Medicine calculation

'Mathematical accuracy is a matter of life and death in clinical nursing' (Keighley, 1984, cited in Cheung, 1986) – an old reference, but certainly one that is still relevant. Drug errors account for 25% of all litigation claims to the NHS (Wright, 2005) and improving the drug calculation skills of nurses is one strategy identified by the Department of Health to try to reduce this number by 40% (Department of Health, 2004). The Department of Health (2004) also states that medication errors are costing the NHS between £200 and £400 million per year.

The *Standards for Medicine Management* (NMC, 2008b, Standard 8) state:

> Some drug administrations can require complex calculations to ensure that the correct volume or quantity of medication is administered. In these situations, it is good practice for a second practitioner (a registered professional) to check the calculation in order to minimise the risk of error. The use of calculators to determine volume or quantity of medication should not act as a substitute for arithmetical knowledge and skill.

## Drug dosages

To calculate drug dosages and intravenous infusion rates requires competence in the use of both fractions and decimals. The formulae suggested are calculated in fractions, while the end result must be in decimals for administration. However, with calculating drugs dosages a certain amount of logic is also required – you should try to predict mentally what the answer is likely to be. For example, the dose ordered is chlorphenamine 3 mg. The stock dose is 2 mg in 5 mL. Is the answer going to be greater or less than 5 mL?

## Fractions

### Simplifying or cancelling down fractions

To simplify a fraction, divide the top and bottom figures by a number that will go into both (a common denominator). For example:

$$\frac{25}{75} = \frac{1}{3} \qquad \text{Both figures have been divided by 25}$$

This calculation may be done in more than one step:

$$\frac{25}{75} \text{ (both divided by 5)} = \frac{5}{15} \text{ (both divided by 5)} = \frac{1}{3}$$

To simplify larger numbers, such as $\frac{800}{1600}$

it is easier to divide the top and bottom figures by 100 (i.e. delete the zeros) leaving

$$\frac{8}{16} = \frac{1}{2}$$

## ACTIVITY 11.5

Simplify the following fractions:

1a $\frac{12}{28}$  1b $\frac{8}{12}$  1c $\frac{75}{150}$  1d $\frac{100}{150}$

1e $\frac{1600}{8000}$  1f $\frac{120}{150}$  1g $\frac{1250}{1600}$  1h $\frac{18}{3}$

Answers to all the activities are at the end of the chapter.

### Changing fractions to decimals

To change a fraction into a decimal, divide the top number by the bottom number. For example:

$$\frac{1}{4} = \text{becomes } 4\overline{)1.00}^{.25}$$

## ACTIVITY 11.6

Change the following to decimals:

2a $\frac{1}{5}$  2b $\frac{1}{2}$  2c $\frac{1}{10}$

## Decimals

Drugs are usually administered in:

- grams (g);

- milligrams (mg);

- micrograms (µg);

- millilitres (ml or mL).

| | | |
|---|---|---|
| 1 kilogram (kg) | = | 1000 grams |
| 1 gram (g) | = | 1000 milligrams |
| 1 milligram (mg) | = | 1000 micrograms |
| 1 litre (l or L) | = | 1000 millilitres |

To carry out drug calculations it may be necessary to convert one unit to another. For example, if the strength of the dose you have is in milligrams, the end calculation must also be in milligrams. Thus, you would first have to convert the dose required to milligrams. *Remember* these units are SI units and therefore always increase or decrease in multiples of 1000.

### *Multiplication of decimals*

Multiplication by 10, 100, 1000, etc. can be done by simply moving the decimal point.

| To multiply by | Move the decimal point |
|---|---|
| 10 | 1 place to the right |
| 100 | 2 places to the right |
| 1000 | 3 places to the right |

For example:

2.0 × 1000 = 2000     Decimal point moved 3 places to the right.

1.3 × 100 = 130     Decimal point moved 2 places to the right.

0.6 × 10 = 6     Decimal point moved 1 place to the right.

---

**ACTIVITY 11.7**

Try the following:

**3a** 0.075 × 10    **3b** 0.003 × 100    **3c** 0.01 × 1000

**3d** 0.2 × 1000    **3e** 0.0505 × 100    **3f** 7.7 × 1000

---

### Division of decimals

To divide decimals by 10, 100, 1000, etc., move the point the other way – to the left.

| To divide by | Move the decimal point |
|---|---|
| 10 | 1 place to the left |
| 100 | 2 places to the left |
| 1000 | 3 places to the left |

For example:

37.8 ÷ 10   = 3.78     Decimal point moved 1 place to the left.

37.8 ÷ 100  = 0.378    Decimal point moved 2 places to the left.

37.8 ÷ 1000 = 0.0378   Decimal point moved 3 places to the left.

## Drug calculation formula

The formula to calculate a dose of medication to be administered is:

$$\frac{\text{what you want}}{\text{what you've got}} \times \frac{\text{what it's in}}{1}$$

For example, if you have 80 mg in 10 mL and you want 200 mg

$$\frac{200}{80} \times \frac{10}{1} = 25 \, \text{mL}$$

As previously stated, it is essential that the units are the same in the calculation. For example, if you have 4 g in 250 mL and you require 800 mg, you need to convert the 4 g to milligrams first before applying the formula:

then 4 g = 4000 mg

$$\frac{800}{4000} \times \frac{250}{1} = 50 \, \text{mL}$$

## ACTIVITY 11.8

Complete these drug calculations:

| Dose ordered | | Stock ampoule / solution |
| --- | --- | --- |
| 4a | ampicillin 350 mg | 500 mg in 100 mL |
| 4b | pethidine 125 mg | 100 mg in 1 mL |
| 4c | phenobarbitone 140 mg | 200 mg in 1 mL |
| 4d | heparin 1250 units | 25000 units in 1 mL |
| 4e | potassium chloride 16 mmol | 26 mmol in 10 mL |
| 4f | digoxin 150 µg | 55 µg in 2 mL |
| 4g | scopolamine 0.3 mg | 0.4 mg in 1 mL |
| 4h | methicillin 1750 mg | 1 g in 2.5 mL |

## Timing the infusion

Intravenous fluids should be prescribed in millilitres, but if they are prescribed in litres this must be converted to millilitres before any calculation can take place.

British Standard adult infusion sets give 15, 20 or 60 drops per mL.

Blood sets     = 15 drops per mL (when blood is transfused)

Solution sets = 20 drops per mL

Burette sets   = 60 drops per mL

The formula to calculate the drops per minute is:

$$\frac{\text{volume of fluid to be infused (in mL)}}{\text{number of hours}} \times \frac{\text{number of drops per mL of giving set}}{60}$$

Round calculations down to the nearest whole number. For example, if 500 mL of Normal Saline is to be infused over 4 hours using a 20 drops per mL set, the rate is:

$$\frac{500}{4} \times \frac{20}{60} = 41 \text{ drops per minute}$$

### ACTIVITY 11.9

Complete the following calculations.

- For a standard 20 drops per mL infusion set, calculate the number of drops per minute to infuse the following:

  **5a**  300 mL over 4 hours        **5b**  145 mL over 1 hour

  **5c**  500 mL over 2.5 hours      **5d**  800 mL over 6 hours

  **5e**  300 mL over 3 hours

- For a blood administration set (15 drops per mL), calculate the following in drops per minute:

  **6a**  150 mL over 2 hours        **6b**  375 mL over 6 hours

  **6c**  225 mL over 3 hours        **6d**  125 mL over 2 hours

  **6e**  165 mL over 2.5 hours

- For a paediatric burette set (60 drops per mL), calculate the drip rates to infuse the following:

  **7a**  320 mL over 4 hours        **7b**  125 mL over 1 hour

  **7c**  250 mL over 4 hours        **7d**  150 mL over 1 hour

  **7e**  50 mL over 30 minutes

# Drug abbreviations

| Abbreviation | English |
|---|---|
| ac | before meals |
| ad lib | freely |
| alte die | alternate days |
| am | morning |
| bid / bd | twice a day |
| c | with |
| cap | capsule |
| ext | external use |
| gtt | drops |
| m | send |
| mg | milligrams |
| ml or mL | millilitres |
| nocte | at night |
| od | once a day |
| o | oral / by mouth |
| pc | after meals |
| pm | evening |
| po | by mouth / oral |
| prn | as needed / required |
| qds | four times a day |
| stat | at once / straight away |
| tab | tablet |
| tds | three times a day |
| top | apply topically to body |

> **FURTHER READING**
>
> *Numeracy, Clinical Calculations and Basic Statistics: A Textbook for Health Care Students* by Neil Davison is a useful guide for nursing students who want to practise and develop their clinical calculation skills.

## Chapter summary

- Student nurses must always be supervised when administering medicines.

- All nurses (including student nurses) must be conversant with the NMC's *Standards for Medicine Management* and the medicine policy of their employer/placement provider (including intravenous policy).

- The '5 rights' must be adhered to when administering medicines.

- Any side-effects of medicines administered or complications of intravenous therapy must be recognised and dealt with appropriately.

## References

Anderson, D., Keith, J. & Novak, P. (2001) *Mosby's Medical, Nursing and Allied Health Dictionary* (6th edition). Amsterdam: Mosby.

Care Standards Act (2000). Available at www.legislation.gov.uk (accessed 14 December 2012)

Cheung, P. (1986) Learning your tables. *Nursing Times*, **82(40)**: 40–41.

Department of Health (2004) *Building a Safer NHS for Patients: Improving Medication Safety*. London: Department of Health.

Dimond, B. (2011) *Legal Aspects of Nursing* (6th edition). London: Pearson.

Dougherty, L. & Lamb, J. (2008) *Intravenous Therapy in Nursing Practice* (2nd edition). Oxford: Blackwell.

Dougherty, L. & Lister, S. (eds) (2011) *The Royal Marsden Hospital Manual of Clinical Nursing Procedures* (8th edition). Oxford: Blackwell.

Gray, A. & Illingworth, J. (2006) *Right Blood, Right Patient, Right Time: RCN Guidance for Improving Transfusion Practice*. London: RCN.

Health Act (2006) Available at www.legislation.gov.uk (accessed 14 December 2012)

Medicinal Products: Prescription by Nurses Act (1992) Available at www.legislation.gov.uk (accessed 20 November 2012)

Medicines Act (1968) Available at www.legislation.gov.uk (accessed 20 November 2012)

Meikle, J. (2000) Parents 'not told' of hospital errors. *The Guardian*, 20 Nov.

Misuse of Drugs Act (1971) Available at www.legislation.gov.uk (accessed 20 November 2012)

Misuse of Drugs Regulations (2001) Available at www.legislation.gov.uk (accessed 20 November 2012)

Misuse of Drugs (Safe Custody) Regulations (1973) Available at www.homeoffice.gov.uk (accessed 14 December 2012)

National Patient Safety Agency (NPSA) (2007) *Promoting Safer Use of Injectable Medicines* (Alert No. 2007/20, 28 March). London: NPSA.

Nursing and Midwifery Council (2007) *Covert Administration of Medicines: Disguising Medicine in Food and Drink* (advice sheet). London: NMC.

Nursing and Midwifery Council (2008a) *The Code: Standards of Conduct, Performance and Ethics for Nurses and Midwives*. London: NMC.

Nursing and Midwifery Council (2008b) *Standards for Medicines Management*. London: NMC.

Peate, I. (2006) *Becoming a Nurse in the 21st Century*. Chichester: Wiley.

Pratt, R., Pellowe, C. Wilson, J. *et al.* (2007) epic2: National evidence-based guidelines for preventing healthcare-associated infections in NHS hospitals in England. *Journal of Hospital Infection*, **65(1):** S1–S12.

Resuscitation Council (UK) (2010) www.resus.org.uk/pages/guide.htm#algos (accessed 20 November 2012)

Royal College of Nursing (2005) *Methicillin-Resistant* Staphylococcus Aureus *(MRSA) Guidance for Nursing Staff.* London: RCN.

The Blood Safety and Quality Regulations (2005) London: HMSO. Available at www.legislation.gov.uk/uksi/2005/50/pdfs/uksi_20050050_en.pdf (accessed 20 November 2012)

Waitt, C., Waitt, P. & Pirmohamed, M. (2004) Intravenous therapy. *Postgraduate Medical Journal,* **(80):** 1–6.

Wright, K. (2005) An exploration into the most effective way to teach drug calculation skills to nursing students. *Nurse Education Today,* **(25):** 430–436.

www.nmc-uk.org (accessed 20 November 2012)

www.rcn.org (accessed 20 November 2012)

www.dh.gov.uk (accessed 20 November 2012)

www.bnf.org (accessed 20 November 2012)

www.resus.org.uk (accessed 20 November 2012)

www.mhra.gov.uk (accessed 20 November 2012)

www.medicines.org.uk/emc (accessed 20 November 2012)

www.npsa.nhs.uk (accessed 20 November 2012)

www.cks.library.nhs.uk/clinical_knowledge/cks-drugs (accessed 20 November 2012)

## Drug calculation answers

| | | | |
|---|---|---|---|
| **1a** $\frac{3}{7}$ | **1b** $\frac{2}{3}$ | **1c** $\frac{1}{2}$ | **1d** $\frac{2}{3}$ |
| **1e** $\frac{1}{5}$ | **1f** $\frac{4}{5}$ | **1g** $\frac{25}{32}$ | **1h** 6 |
| **2a** 0.2 | **2b** 0.5 | **2c** 0.1 | |
| **3a** 0.75 | **3b** 0.3 | **3c** 10 | **3d** 200 |
| **3e** 5.05 | **3f** 7700 | | |
| **4a** 70 mL | **4b** 1.25 mL | **4c** 0.7 mL | **4d** 0.05 mL |

**4e** 6.15 mL          **4f** 5.45 mL          **4g** 0.75 mL          **4h** 4.38 mL

## Infusion rate answers

**5a** 25          **5b** 48          **5c** 66          **5d** 44          **5e** 33

**6a** 18          **6b** 15          **6c** 18          **6d** 15          **6e** 16

**7a** 80          **7b** 125          **7c** 62          **7d** 150          **7e** 100

# INDEX